Current Concepts in Cariology

Guest Editors

DOUGLAS A. YOUNG, DDS, MS, MBA
MARGHERITA FONTANA, DDS, PhD
MARK S. WOLFF, DDS, PhD

DENTAL CLINICS OF NORTH AMERICA

www.dental.theclinics.com

July 2010 • Volume 54 • Number 3

SAUNDERS an imprint of ELSEVIER, Inc.

W.B. SAUNDERS COMPANY
A Division of Elsevier Inc.

1600 John F. Kennedy Boulevard ● Suite 1800 ● Philadelphia, Pennsylvania 19103-2899

http://www.dental.theclinics.com

DENTAL CLINICS OF NORTH AMERICA Volume 54, Number 3
July 2010 ISSN 0011-8532, ISBN-978-1-4377-2440-0

Editor: John Vassallo; j.vassallo@elsevier.com

Dental Clinics of North America (ISSN 0011-8532) is published quarterly by Elsevier Inc., 360 Park Avenue South, New York, NY 10010-1710. Months of issue are January, April, July, and October. Business and Editorial Offices: 1600 John F. Kennedy Boulevard, Suite 1800, Philadelphia, PA 19103-2899. Periodicals postage paid at New York, NY and additional mailing offices. Subscription prices are $224.00 per year (domestic individuals), $382.00 per year (domestic institutions), $108.00 per year (domestic students/residents), $266.00 per year (Canadian individuals), $481.00 per year (Canadian institutions), $321.00 per year (international individuals), $481.00 per year (international institutions), and $162.00 per year (international and Canadian students/residents). International air speed delivery is included in all *Clinics* subscription prices. All prices are subject to change without notice. **POSTMASTER:** Send address changes to *Dental Clinics of North America*, Elsevier Health Sciences Division, Subscription Customer Service, 3251 Riverport Lane, Maryland Heights, MO 63043. **Customer Service (orders, claims, online, change of address): Elsevier Health Sciences Division, Subscription Customer Service, 3251 Riverport Lane, Maryland Heights, MO 63043. Tel: 1-800-654-2452 (U.S. and Canada). Fax: 314-447-8029. E-mail: journalscustomerservice-usa@elsevier.com (for print support); journalsonlinesupport-usa@elsevier.com (for online support).**

Reprints. For copies of 100 or more, of articles in this publication, please contact the Commercial Reprints Department, Elsevier Inc., 360 Park Avenue South, New York, NY 10010-1710. Tel.: 212-633-3812; Fax: 212-462-1935; E-mail: reprints@elsevier.com.

The *Dental Clinics of North America* is covered in *MEDLINE/PubMed (Index Medicus), Current Contents/Clinical Medicine, ISI/BIOMED* and *Clinahl*.

Printed in the United States of America.

Contributors

GUEST EDITORS

DOUGLAS A. YOUNG, DDS, MS, MBA
Associate Professor, Department of Dental Practice, University of the Pacific, Arthur A. Dugoni School of Dentistry, San Francisco, California

MARGHERITA FONTANA, DDS, PhD
Associate Professor, Department of Cariology, Restorative Sciences and Endodontics, University of Michigan School of Dentistry, Ann Arbor, Michigan

MARK S. WOLFF, DDS, PhD
Professor and Chair, Department of Cariology and Comprehensive Care, New York University College of Dentistry, New York, New York

AUTHORS

MARIANA M. BRAGA, DDS, PhD
Department of Pediatric Dentistry, Faculdade de Odontologia da Universidade de São Paulo, Avenida Professor Lineu Prestes, São Paulo, Brazil

KIM R. EKSTRAND, DDS, PhD
Department of Cariology and Endodontics, School of Dentistry, Faculty of Health Sciences, University of Copenhagen, Copenhagen, Denmark

JOHN D.B. FEATHERSTONE, MSc, PhD
Professor and Dean, University of California, San Francisco, School of Dentistry, San Francisco, California

MARGHERITA FONTANA, DDS, PhD
Associate Professor, Department of Cariology, Restorative Sciences and Endodontics, University of Michigan School of Dentistry, Ann Arbor, Michigan

CARLOS GONZÁLEZ-CABEZAS, DDS, MSD, PhD
Associate Professor, Department of Cariology, Restorative Sciences, and Endodontics, University of Michigan School of Dentistry, Ann Arbor, Michigan

ANDERSON T. HARA, DDS, MS, PhD
Assistant Professor, Department of Preventive and Community Dentistry, Indiana University School of Dentistry, Indianapolis, Indiana

EDWINA A.M. KIDD, BDS, FDSRCS, PhD, DSc Med
Emerita Professor of Cariology, Kings College London, England, United Kingdom

CHRIS LONGBOTTOM, BDS, PhD
Senior Lecturer and Associate Director, Dental Health Services and Research Unit, Centre for Clinical Innovations, University of Dundee, Dundee, Scotland, United Kingdom

ADRIAN LUSSI, Ms of Chem DMD, PhD
Professor, Department of Preventive, Restorative and Pediatric Dentistry, School of Dental Medicine, University of Bern, Bern, Switzerland

PHILIP D. MARSH, PhD
Professor, Health Protection Agency, Centre for Emergency Preparedness and Response, Salisbury; Department of Oral Biology, Leeds Dental Institute, Leeds, United Kingdom

FAUSTO M. MENDES, DDS, MS, PhD
Department of Pediatric Dentistry, Faculdade de Odontologia da Universidade de São Paulo, Avenida Professor Lineu Prestes, São Paulo, Brazil

HIEN NGO, BDS, MDS, PhD, FADI, FICD, FPFA
Professor, Chair, General Dental Practice, School of Dentistry, The University of Queensland, Queensland, Australia

MATHILDE C. PETERS, DMD, PhD
Professor of Dentistry, Department of Cariology, Restorative Sciences and Endodontics, University of Michigan School of Dentistry, Ann Arbor, Michigan

NIGEL B. PITTS, BDS, PhD, FDS, FFGDP, FFPH, FRSE
Professor and Director, Dental Health Services and Research Unit, Centre for Clinical Innovations, University of Dundee, Dundee, Scotland, United Kingdom

SVANTE TWETMAN, DDS, Odont Dr
Professor of Cariology, Department of Cariology and Endodontics, Institute of Odontology, Faculty of Health Sciences, University of Copenhagen, Denmark; Director, Maxillofacial Unit, County Hospital, Halmstad, Sweden

XIAOJIE WANG, DMD, PhD
Department of Preventive, Restorative and Pediatric Dentistry, School of Dental Medicine, University of Bern, Bern, Switzerland

MARK S. WOLFF, DDS, PhD
Professor and Chair, Department of Cariology and Comprehensive Care, New York University College of Dentistry, New York, New York

DOUGLAS A. YOUNG, DDS, MS, MBA
Associate Professor, Department of Dental Practice, University of the Pacific, Author A. Dugoni School of Dentistry, San Francisco, California

DOMENICK T. ZERO, DDS, MS
Professor, Department of Preventive and Community Dentistry, Indiana University School of Dentistry, Indianapolis, Indiana

Contents

> This introductory article provides an overview of the caries disease pro-
> cess that will help guide readers into the world of evidence-based caries
> management in the beginning of the twenty-first century and help them un-
> derstand the ongoing need to update in this field. This issue of *Dental
> Clinics of North America* provides clinically relevant reviews, full of chair-
> side recommendations based on best available evidence, on epidemiol-
> ogy, nomenclature, disease process, and management. A glossary of
> common terms in cariology is included.

> Dental plaque is the biofilm found naturally on teeth. Dental plaque is also
> implicated in dental caries, which is associated with shifts in the microbial
> balance of the biofilm resulting in increased proportions of acid producing
> and acid tolerating bacteria, especially (but not exclusively) mutans strep-
> tococci and lactobacilli. The regular intake of fermentable dietary sugars,
> or impaired saliva flow, produces persistent conditions of low pH within
> the biofilm, which selects for these cariogenic bacteria. Clinicians should
> prevent this disruption to the natural microbial balance of the biofilm (rel-
> evant approaches are described) rather than merely treating its conse-
> quences by restoring cavities.

> The pathogenicity of the dental biofilm is modified by salivary and dietary
> factors, as well as by the characteristics of the tooth structure. The com-
> position of the acquired pellicle can modify the mineral homeostasis of the
> tooth surfaces and the attachment of bacteria for the development of the
> biofilm. The substitution of sucrose from the diet by other less cariogenic
> sugars and/or sugar substitutes can contribute to reducing the pathoge-
> nicity of the biofilm. Saliva clears, dilutes, neutralizes, and buffers acids
> produced by the biofilm. In addition, saliva provides the biofilm/tooth
> structure with Ca^{2+} PO_4^{3-} and F^- ions, which can positively affect the

arrest, and remineralize caries lesions. With the rapidly increasing knowledge about oral biofilms and the process of caries in itself, the profession is embarking on new strategies. This is an exciting time, with several promising new agents and novel treatment modalities at the horizon to prevent and manage caries lesions. Some are already available in clinical practice. Studies, however, have yet to show conclusive evidence of clinical efficacy. None have shown to be more effective than fluoride and protection by sealant.

This article reviews the evidence for saliva diagnostics and some antibacterial concepts with potential to interfere with the caries process. It concludes that there is incomplete evidence to evaluate the role of chairside tests and to recommend general topical applications of antibacterial agents to prevent caries lesions. However, such measures may be considered to control the disease in caries-active individuals. There is evidence that xylitol has antibacterial properties that alter the oral ecology but the clinical evidence for caries prevention is rated as fair. However, preventive programs should include as many complementary strategies as possible, especially when directed toward caries-active patients. Therefore, any antibacterial intervention should always be combined with a fluoride program, until stronger evidence for its use in caries prevention and management becomes available.

There would appear to be little logic in the current practice of caries removal. Biologically, it would appear to be potentially damaging even to attempt to remove all infected dentin in a symptomless, vital tooth. It is neither possible nor necessary to achieve this. The evidence would seem to show that, provided a restoration is placed that seals the cavity, infected dentin may be left. It does not prejudice pulpal health, and the caries lesion does not progress.

This article focuses on glass-ionomer cement (GIC) and its role in the clinical management of caries. It begins with a brief description of GIC, the mechanism of fluoride release and ion exchange, the interaction between GIC and the external environment, and finally the ion exchange between GIC and the tooth at the internal interface. The importance of GIC, as a tool, in caries management, in minimal intervention dentistry (MI), and Caries Management by Risk Assessment (CAMBRA) also will be highlighted.

Studies have shown a growing trend toward increasing prevalence of dental erosion, associated with the declining prevalence of caries disease in industrialized countries. Erosion is an irreversible chemical process that results in tooth substance loss and leaves teeth susceptible to damage as a result of wear over the course of an individual's lifetime. Therefore, early diagnosis and adequate prevention are essential to minimize the risk of tooth erosion. Clinical appearance is the most important sign to be used to diagnose erosion. The Basic Erosive Wear Examination (BEWE) is a simple method to fulfill this task. The determination of a variety of risk and protective factors (patient-dependent and nutrition-dependent factors) as well as their interplay are necessary to initiate preventive measures tailored to the individual. When tooth loss caused by erosive wear reaches a certain level, oral rehabilitation becomes necessary.

THE CLINICS ARE NOW AVAILABLE ONLINE!

Access your subscription at:
www.theclinics.com

Dedication

We dedicate this issue to our friend and mentor, John Featherstone, as it was he who brought each of us together to collaborate several years ago, which led to many advancements in caries management and ultimately this publication.

Douglas A. Young

Margherita Fontana

Mark S. Wolff

E-mail addresses:
dyoung@pacific.edu (D.A. Young)
mfontan@umich.edu (M. Fontana)
mark.wolff@nyu.edu (M.S. Wolff)

Dent Clin N Am 54 (2010) xi
doi:10.1016/j.cden.2010.04.004
0011-8532/10/$ – see front matter © 2010 Elsevier Inc. All rights reserved.

Preface

Current Concepts in Cariology

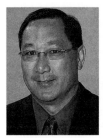 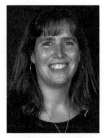 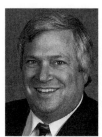

Douglas A. Young, DDS, MS, MBA

Margherita Fontana, DDS, PhD

Mark S. Wolff, DDS, PhD

Guest Editors

The evolution of a paradigm shift may take decades and usually involves several stake-holders.[1,2] In the case of caries management by risk assessment (CAMBRA), the main premise is based on the fact that traditional restorative repair of teeth did little to treat the actual cause and risk factors of the disease; thus, by using CAMBRA principles it is possible to assess the risk of individual patients and establish evidence-based management strategies based on that risk. For several decades the role of bacteria and the chemistry of the remineralization-demineralization process were well understood, yet the scientific evidence alone did not result in significant change in clinical practice.

CAMBRA GAINS MOMENTUM THROUGH COLLABORATION

In 2002, John Featherstone and Douglas Young decided to establish an interorganizational collaborative, which included members from education, research, industry, governmental agencies, and private practitioners based in the Western United States.[3] This unofficial group was called the Western CAMBRA Coalition and proved successful in advancing the CAMBRA paradigm. For example, in 2003, the science of CAMBRA was published in the February and March issues of the *Journal of the California Dental Association*. The collaboration led to sharing of information between dental schools so that in short order all Western schools were teaching CAMBRA in their curricula. At the same time, members of the collaborative helped implement a $7 million First 5 grant to educate medical and dental providers in California on this new method of prevention and treatment of dental caries disease. In 2007, the *Journal of the California Dental Association* devoted another two journal issues to the clinical implementation of CAMBRA, including example protocols.[4,5] For the first time, an example protocol was presented so that clinical practices could have a starting point to implement CAMBRA in actual

Dent Clin N Am 54 (2010) xiii–xv
doi:10.1016/j.cden.2010.04.003
0011-8532/10/$ – see front matter © 2010 Elsevier Inc. All rights reserved.

practice. In November 2007, the California Dental Association House of Delegates adopted a resolution to support the core principles of the CAMBRA consensus statement published in the *Journal of the California Dental Association* that same month. The adoption established the CAMBRA principles as policy for the California Dental Association. The four journals can be accessed at www.cdafoundation.org/journal.

The success of collaboration was then leveraged nationally by the formation of the Central CAMBRA Coalition, led by Margherita Fontana, and the Eastern CAMBRA Coalition, led by Mark Wolff. Together these three unofficial groups were able to catapult CAMBRA principles into mainstream US education by the formation of a new cariology section in 2010 within the American Dental Education Association (ADEA). On March 3, 2010, the ADEA House of Delegates adopted a resolution to support the core principles of CAMBRA as policy.

CURRENT TEXT NEEDED

Despite the progress CAMBRA has made in recent years, it still falls short of inclusion in mainstream practice. The behavior of the profession must shift from a surgical-only approach to caries management toward a system that science demonstrates has clear advantages over traditional methods. The science has progressed in all areas of CAMBRA and there is a great need for a single text that targets practicing clinicians and students who have not yet been exposed to CAMBRA from other sources.

A PREVIEW OF THIS ISSUE

This issue begins by discussing the different levels of scientific evidence and accepted terminology as they relate to current understanding of the caries disease process. The scientific levels of evidence for these new innovative CAMBRA treatments also vary. Recent attention to evidence-based clinical treatments have led to the distinction between those interventions used for primary caries disease prevention and those used for already existing disease (secondary disease prevention). Revolutionary new theories on the effect of the oral environment on the way biofilm will ultimately behave (acid producing or not) are presented. No longer is the disease blamed on just a few causative agents but rather attention is drawn toward the role of the environment and how a drop in pH in the environment can cause a pathologic shift in the biofilm. The interaction of saliva, pellicle, diet, and hard tissue ultrastructure also is a key determinant of whether or not demineralization or remineralization will ultimately predominate. Subsequent articles provide updates on the latest information on the detection and diagnosis of caries lesions. Caries risk assessment will be taught as a method to determine which factors are increasing the chance of demineralization on a given individual so that intervening strategies may be implemented to halt or reverse disease. The latest science on noninvasive chemical repair methodologies as well as minimally invasive biocompatible dental materials are reviewed. Readers will know when to treat chemically and when to treat surgically as well as how much and what type of tooth mineral must be removed during surgical preparation for restorative procedures. Finally there is a review on nonbacterial erosive damage to teeth.

THE HOPE

The scientific principles of CAMBRA have initiated a paradigm shift in the way caries disease is managed around the world, with many of the advances coming from other countries. This edition of *Dental Clinics of North America* has been successful in attracting the leading experts from around the globe in all aspects of this multifactorial disease process. It is our sincere hope that this issue gives students and practicing clinicians the most current perspective on treating dental caries disease. By using the best available science to supplement (not replace) the highest levels of evidence (fluoride and sealants), we will be one more step closer to promoting oral health and thus overall health as well as addressing the access to care issues worldwide. Patients are the first to notice and appreciate the shift toward disease treatment and disease prevention rather than waiting for disease to cause significant damage to teeth that requires surgical restorative repair. Another key to successful implementation of CAMBRA into mainstream clinical practice is the development of a solid economic model.

We hope that after reading this text the decision to implement the science presented can be answered based on two questions:

1. Does the CAMBRA paradigm have a relative advantage for patients over the current surgical-only model?
2. If so, is there an ethical obligation to change?

Douglas A. Young, DDS, MS, MBA
Department of Dental Practice
University of the Pacific, Arthur A. Dugoni School of Dentistry
2155 Webster Street, Room 400
San Francisco, CA 94115, USA

Margherita Fontana, DDS, PhD
Department of Cariology, Restorative Sciences and Endodontics
University of Michigan School of Dentistry
1011 North University, Room 2029b
Ann Arbor, MI 48109-1078, USA

Mark S. Wolff, DDS, PhD
Department of Cariology and Comprehensive Care
New York University College of Dentistry
345 East 24th Street (MC9480)
New York, NY 10010, USA

E-mail addresses:
dyoung@pacific.edu (D.A. Young)
mfontan@umich.edu (M. Fontana)
mark.wolff@nyu.edu (M.S. Wolff)

REFERENCES

1. Kuhn T. The structure of scientific revolutions. 3rd edition. Chicago: University of Chicago Press; 1996.
2. Rogers E. Diffusion of innovations. New York: Free Press; 2003.
3. Young DA, Buchanan PM, Lubman RG, et al. New directions in interorganizational collaboration in dentistry: the CAMBRA Coalition model. J Dent Educ 2007;71(5):595–600.
4. Jenson L, Budenz AW, Featherstone JD, et al. Clinical protocols for caries management by risk assessment. J Calif Dent Assoc 2007;35(10):714–23.
5. Ramos-Gomez FJ, Crall J, Gansky SA, et al. Caries risk assessment appropriate for the age 1 visit (infants and toddlers). J Calif Dent Assoc 2007;35(10):687–702.

Defining Dental Caries for 2010 and Beyond

Margherita Fontana, DDS, PhD[a],*, Douglas A. Young, DDS, MS, MBA[b],
Mark S. Wolff, DDS, PhD[c], Nigel B. Pitts, BDS, PhD, FDS, FFGDP, FFPH, FRSE[d],
Chris Longbottom, BDS, PhD[d]

KEYWORDS

- Dental caries • Definitions • Terminology • Glossary
- Evidence base

The objective of this introductory article is to provide an overview of the caries disease process that will help guide the readers into the world of evidence-based caries management in the beginning of the 21st century and help them understand the need to keep updating in this field. This issue of the *Dental Clinics of North America* provides clinically relevant reviews, full of chair-side recommendations based on best available evidence, of the etiologic drivers of the caries process, starting with its microbiology (Marsh), the role of environmental drivers such as saliva, pellicle, diet, and hard tissue ultrastructure (Hara and Zero), how to understand normal versus abnormal demineralization-remineralization (Gonzalez-Cabezas), how to best detect and diagnose caries lesions (Braga and colleagues), moving to very practical recommendations on how to assess patients' risk (Young and Featherstone), what strategies are available for noninvasive demineralized tissue repair (Peters), existing treatment protocols for the management of the disease process (Twetman), evidence to support thresholds for partial or complete caries removal (Kidd), how to do minimally invasive dentistry taking advantage of bioactive restorative materials (Ngo), and finally, addressing dental erosion, an emerging relevant problem that has many similarities with dental caries but also many differences in its clinical management (Wang and Lussi).

[a] Department of Cariology, Restorative Sciences and Endodontics, University of Michigan School of Dentistry, 1011 n University Avenue, Ann Arbor, MI 48109, USA
[b] Department of Dental Practice, University of the Pacific, Arthur A. Dugoni School of Dentistry, 2155 Webster Street, Room 400, San Francisco, CA 94115, USA
[c] Department of Cariology and Comprehensive Care, New York University College of Dentistry, 345 East 24th Street (MC9480), New York, NY 10010, USA
[d] Dental Health Services & Research Unit, Centre for Clinical Innovations, University of Dundee, Mackenzie Building, Kirsty Semple Way, Dundee DD2 4BF, Scotland, UK
* Corresponding author.
E-mail address: mfontan@umich.edu

Dent Clin N Am 54 (2010) 423–440
doi:10.1016/j.cden.2010.03.007
0011-8532/10/$ – see front matter © 2010 Elsevier Inc. All rights reserved.

EPIDEMIOLOGY

Although significant caries prevalence has been noted since the time of pre-Neolithic humans (10,000 BC) with reported caries prevalence between 1.4% and 12.1% carious teeth, it was not until the fourteenth and fifteenth century when a sharp increase in caries prevalence was noted. This increase is often ascribed to a sucrose-civilization-caries trinity, with caries prevalence rising above 25%. The sucrose-civilization-caries trinity fails to describe the entire picture. At the same time as sucrose consumption increased, so did life expectancy.[1] These observations hold true today as the world's population continues to grow older, retaining teeth longer. Worldwide caries prevalence varies widely. Caries prevalence is generally reported as decayed-missing-filled teeth (DMFT) or decayed-missing-filled surfaces (DMFS). Caries prevalence estimates have been most frequently based on caries visibly (or occasionally also using radiographs) penetrating to the dento-enamel junction (the so-called D_3MF, dentinal caries diagnostic threshold). Dental caries and tooth loss were among the most common causes for rejection from service in the American Civil War and both World Wars.[2] With the introduction of fluoride, both in the public water supply and toothpaste, a change in the worldwide ubiquitous nature of dental caries occurred. Nations and individuals with the financial resources available to invest in oral health have seen steep improvements in both DMFS and DMFT during the latter half of the twentieth century. As examples, mean DMFT in all age groups in the United States has decreased from 38.30 DMFS to 27.86 DMFS during the interval 1971 to 2005[3] with the most significant improvements in children younger than 12 years.[4] Socio-economic status and level of education are key factors, both at the individual and national levels. A study in Scotland on 5-year-old children demonstrated a direct relationship between the number of untreated decayed surfaces and filled teeth with social deprivation.[5] An analysis of data in the United States reveals that adults are 4 times more likely to be edentulous if they have not graduated from high school or live below the federal poverty level.[2] Industrialized countries with high gross domestic product (GDP) have recognized a significant reduction in DMFT while countries with medium GDP per capita have the highest DMFT. Countries with the lowest GDP actually have the lowest DMFT in 12-year-olds, which may reflect a financial inability of families to purchase large amounts of processed sucrose-containing foods.[6] Socio-economic conditions affect caries rates throughout the world but are not the only determinant of caries prevalence, as demonstrated by the prevalence of caries in 5- to 7-year-old children throughout Europe. Children's caries prevalence ranged from less than 1 decayed and filled tooth in Ireland (east) to 5.5 decayed and filled teeth in Poland.[7]

Epidemiologic study of caries distribution also reflects the change in population demographics. For instance, a 2005 report on caries in the United States revealed that 31% of adults older than 60 years had root caries (treated and restored) whereas the presence of root caries was less than 9% in those younger than 40. Although the number of adults older than 60 years had increased since 1988, so also did the number of adults older than 60 who retained their teeth. Significant progress has been achieved in preventing caries in the younger population but disease trends internationally indicate that the prevalence of caries in later adulthood remains significant, with 91% of dentate adults older than 20 years having caries experience.[2] In addition to increases in root caries seen with aging, as populations have seen decreases in caries from the introduction of fluoride, the decrease in caries has not been evenly distributed over all surfaces of the teeth. Significant reductions in smooth-surface caries have been noted with the introduction of fluoride in both public water supply and toothpaste, but commensurate reductions in occlusal caries have not been seen as the result from fluoride. Additional preventive strategies are required.

All of the above trends and research reflect a bias toward surgical dental care where surgical intervention is required when caries reaches the dento-enamel junction. As subsequent articles describe, the dental caries process starts long before the cavitation is noted. Further, new criteria for detection (as discussed later) and new mechanisms of treatment mandate a "new" definition of caries. This "new" definition, reflected in all the articles of this issue, leads to the determination that the prevalence of caries disease may be much greater because the detection criteria were so crude in looking for signs of cavitation rather than the earlier signs of demineralization, which may be reversible and preventable with the current therapies. As stated by Pitts and colleagues in 2003,[8] "where data are collected and reported at the D_3 (caries into dentin only) threshold, the proportion of the population classified as 'caries free' conveys the mistaken impression that there is no disease at all present...." Internationally, epidemiologic assessments of caries prevalence are increasingly being undertaken at the D_1 (caries into enamel and/or dentin threshold) to capture more of the true caries burden.[8]

THE ISSUE WITH NOMENCLATURE

One of the recurring themes of this review is the need for recording of caries lesion severity and activity in our clinical charts as a starting point to risk assessment and monitoring of the impact of management strategies aiming to control the caries disease process and arrest or remineralize caries lesions. Thus, it would seem logical that the discussion should begin with a critical review of nomenclature and its importance in driving diagnostic and management strategies, including a definition of dental caries and a glossary of commonly used terms in cariology. As simple as this task seems to be, it is evident that one of the major barriers in the translation of caries detection, assessment, diagnosis, risk assessment, and management findings from the research domain to everyday clinical practice has been the confusion around the variety of terms clinical dentistry, education, and research choose to use when referring to dental caries. Warren wrote a very provocative editorial in the *Journal of Operative Dentistry* (1998) called "Coming to Terms with Terminology."[9] In it, he suggested that "accuracy of definition and use of terms is essential to clear thinking and communication." In fact, the way we choose to communicate may reflect what we believe or understand regarding the caries process and hence, how we eventually choose to act. As stated so elegantly by the International Caries Detection and Assessment System (ICDAS) Coordinating Committee[10] (www. ICDAS.org), "the future of research, practice, and education in cariology requires the development of an integrated definition of dental caries and uniform systems for measuring the caries process." This is important not only for communications between clinicians to accurately take place, but it is also essential for accurate communication with patients.[11] Several consensus development conferences, committees, and dental organizations have addressed this problem in recent years by debating and developing definitions which reflect up-to-date evidence in relation to various specific key aspects of caries.[11] Our goal will be merely to highlight some of those, adding to them when necessary, to fuel this constructive discussion and clarification process. At the end of this article we have included a glossary of terms in cariology, with references to appropriate sources, starting with the most current glossary published by Longbottom and colleagues in 2009,[11] which included representatives of the ICDAS, the European Organization for Caries Research (ORCA), the European Association of Dental Public Health (EADPH), and the American Dental Education Association (ADEA) Cariology Special Interest Group (SIG, now Section). This glossary has also been distributed internationally as an early part of the FDI World Dental Federation's Global Caries Initiative, in response to the expressed need from the launch event for a common language to discuss modern cariology and preventive caries care. We also include, when appropriate, a discussion of terms commonly used in practice in North America that have in some instances hampered, and in other instances complicated the translation of best evidence into best practice.

Dental caries is the localized destruction of susceptible dental hard tissue by acidic by-products from bacterial fermentation of dietary carbohydrates.[11] If allowed to progress the disease will result in the development of detectable changes in the tooth structure, or caries lesions,[12] which initially are noncavitated (ie, macroscopically intact), but which eventually might progress to cavitation. Dental caries is not the "cavity" in the tooth,[13] therefore, we cannot "remove all the caries."[9] The "medical model," where the etiologic disease-driving agents are balanced against protective factors, in combination with risk assessment,[14,15] offers the possibility of patient-centered disease prevention and management before there is irreversible damage done to the teeth.[16,17] In 2001, the NIH Consensus Development Conference on Diagnosis and Management of Dental Caries Throughout Life identified the need to use new strategies "to provide enhanced access for those who suffer disproportionately from the disease; to provide improved detection, risk assessment, and diagnosis; and to create—and enhance use of—improved methods to arrest or reverse the non-cavitated lesion while improving surgical management of the cavitated lesion."[18] If one does not start by differentiating between the caries disease process and the caries lesion, and focus only on the cavity, the need for disease management and remineralization is de-emphasized.

Furthermore, in dentistry the terms caries diagnosis and caries detection are very often used incorrectly and interchangeably. This usage is possibly due to the fact that the earlier stages of the disease process are virtually symptom-free, giving the perception by many, in the restorative dominated strategies of the past, that a diagnostic step is not needed,[19,20] and that caries assessment becomes ultimately a question of detection, that is, whether caries lesions are present or not. Furthermore, the detection of frank cavitations in teeth requiring restoration is still considered by many as the main focus of caries treatment plans. By contrast, modern dental caries management should focus on the detection of earlier stages of the disease process (eg, noncavitated caries lesions) and the practitioner's ability to diagnose whether those lesions are active, in addition to the identification and assessment of more severe lesions. An International Consensus Workshop on Caries Clinical Trials (ICW-CCT) was held in 2002 involving 95 participants from 23 countries. The final Consensus Statements represent international agreement on where the evidence leads in caries clinical trials,[12] and in it important definitions of caries detection, assessment, and diagnosis were provided. To "diagnose" dental caries implies not only an objective determination of whether lesion(s) or disease is present at one point in time (ie, detection), and a characterization of how severe it is once it has been detected (ie, caries assessment) but, most importantly, assimilation by a human professional of all available data to decide if it is active or arrested. This diagnosis should be one of the guiding factors for caries risk assessment (risk of developing new lesions in the future[21]) and management (encompassing surgical and nonsurgical care and prevention), and decision making.[12,21,22]

To apply these concepts we must start by deciding what we need to record in our clinical settings and what we should call each element. Based on current thinking, certainly a continuous measure of lesion severity and activity is required to help guide the diagnostic and monitoring steps.[13,17] We further propose that we set as a goal the elimination in our daily lexicon of terms that are not diagnostic (eg, that the patient is "caries free" when a full examination of clean dry teeth with the benefit of lesion detection aids has not been performed, or "the patient has a decalcification") or terms that merely reflect uncertainty in the diagnosis (eg, this is a "watch"). Without undertaking a diagnostic decision as to whether a lesion is active, be it progressing slowly or rapidly, or arrested, a logical clinical treatment decision cannot be made.[22] Of utmost importance is to clearly define lesion thresholds and clinical conditions that separate surgical from nonsurgical interventions, as these have immediate treatment consequences. As an example, an international effort has created a new set of harmonized criteria building on best evidence,[23] ICDAS[10] (www.ICDAS.org), designed to be a unifying, predominantly visual set of criteria codes based on the characteristics of clean, dry teeth at both the enamel and dentin caries levels, which is capable of assessing both caries severity and activity, and has supporting histologic validation.[24–27] For clarity, the shared aim of the ICDAS initiative, which drives the focus on agreed definitions for the "stages" of caries, are that ICDAS is: (a) a clinical visual caries scoring system for use in clinical practice, dental education, research, and epidemiology, (b) designed to lead to better-quality information to inform decisions about appropriate diagnosis, prognosis, and clinical management at both the individual and public health levels, and (c) the provider of a framework to support and enable personalized comprehensive caries management for improved long-term health outcomes.[28]

HOW ABOUT EVIDENCE-BASED DENTISTRY AND CARIES MANAGEMENT?

The more traditional methods used for treating dental caries in practice today remain largely focused on the use of surgical tooth restoration alone (ie, restorative treatment), without consistent and individualized consideration of the underlying disease process for each patient. However, there is limited evidence that restorative care is effective in preventing or managing the dental caries disease process in the longer term. Clinical trials that provide clear evidence regarding the effectiveness of various interventions are, as yet, insufficient to permit the formulation of definitive guidelines for all cases. Thus, the clinician is left with two choices: (1) to continue using the outdated traditional restorative-only approach based on irreversible procedures, or (2) to use nondestructive risk-based caries management strategies using the best scientific evidence available. The latter choice is the one that the scientific and best practice clinical community has been encouraging the profession to embrace on a national and international level.[29] Apart from fluorides and sealants, highest-quality evidence for other therapeutic caries management strategies is limited and contentious, and so dentists are encouraged not to incorporate these strategies as a replacement of higher-evidence strategies, but rather as supplements to them, if so desired. It is clear that the search for more effective and practical therapeutic approaches for the management of patients at risk of dental caries needs to continue, as does the search for stronger evidence for available treatment strategies/choices. As new evidence appears and is assessed, caries management strategies need to be able to evolve without decades of delay or the impairment of remuneration systems. In summary, the goal of ideal evidence-based patient care is to always select the therapeutic option that is supported by the highest level of evidence, and is practicable, feasible, and acceptable to the particular dentist-patient team.[16] As we move forward in caries detection, assessment, and preventive management, we should continue to be guided by an evidence-based dentistry philosophy to plan care that results in *doing the right thing, done right, at the right time for the right person.* For this reason there is an increasing focus on patient-centered, personalized treatment plans, rather than a traditional mechanistic focus in which very different patients with different states of disease activity, caries risk, behaviors, and needs end up with very similar "automatic" care plans.[28]

AN OVERVIEW AND UPDATE OF THE CARIES DISEASE PROCESS: PRELUDE TO THE ARTICLES THAT FOLLOW

The etiology of caries disease is certainly multifactorial; however, the presence of an acidogenic bacterial biofilm is an absolute requirement for bacterial acid generation. We now know that dental caries disease is a transmissible infection that can be treated and even prevented before damage to dental hard tissue occurs. Recent research has challenged the concept of mutans streptococci and lactobacilli as the only important bacteria in caries disease. Article by Philip D. Marsh elsewhere in this issue examines the complexities of oral biofilms, where multiple bacterial species interact in a dynamic environment. In this environment, pH fluctuations result in large ecological changes, with an acidic environment driving selection of a cariogenic biofilm. However, an acidogenic biofilm is not the only factor that determines caries disease activity; environmental factors such as saliva, pellicle, diet, and hard tissue ultrastructure all are critical. Article by Hara and Zero elsewhere in this issue examines the role of each environmental factor in relation to caries disease. However, remineralization and demineralization of dental hard tissues depends on the dynamic chemistry within the oral cavity. This dynamic process of demineralization and remineralization occurs often throughout the day. As long as there is not a net mineral loss, there will be no permanent changes to the tooth and the process is considered to be in a healthy balanced state; this is reviewed in detail in the article by Carlos González-Cabezas elsewhere in this issue. However, when there is a net mineral loss from the tooth then a caries lesion will develop or an existing lesion will progress. Detecting and diagnosing caries lesions at the earliest possible stage are the key to chemically arresting and reversing the demineralization process, and are discussed in the article by Braga and colleagues elsewhere in this issue. If demineralization and remineralization occurs on all individuals, why do some people get caries lesions while others do not? This question is answered in the article by Young and Featherstone elsewhere in this issue by the caries balance/imbalance concept[14] whereby pathologic caries risk factors and disease indicators are balanced against the protective factors. By evaluating the current caries risk of a patient, a clinician can determine what behaviors are increasing a patient's risk for disease and disease progression, and take corrective action. These strategies lead to the development of evidence-based questionnaires or caries risk assessment forms to help determine caries risk and to suggest effective treatment options based on that risk. Using this new protocol it has become possible to develop a treatment plan designed to arrest dental caries by stopping demineralization, or reverse the caries disease process via remineralization, therefore reducing the chance of cavitation. This process has been called caries management by risk assessment (CAMBRA).

Article by Mathilde C. Peters elsewhere in this issue reviews suggestions for noninvasive repair of demineralized, precavitated (no-cavitated) lesions. The art of CAMBRA comes into play when the clinician must find ways to educate and motivate patients to change the pathologic behaviors identified by the caries risk assessment. While reading the article by Mathilde C. Peters elsewhere in this issue, keep in mind that there are many ways (rather than one correct way) and increasing numbers of products to assist in rebalancing the patient's oral health. Article by Mathilde C. Peters elsewhere in this issue reviews what strategies are available for noninvasive demineralized tissue repair, while the article by Svante Twetman elsewhere in this issue reviews existing treatment protocols for the management of the disease process. Article by Edwina A.M. Kidd elsewhere in this issue reviews guidelines on when to restore surgically (compared with chemical remineralization). The evidence to support thresholds for partial or complete caries removal is presented. When continued removal of the remaining infected dentin is very likely to lead to pulp exposure on an asymptomatic vital tooth, the concept of sealing in active demineralization is discussed. In addition, the research demonstrating that stain does not correlate to bacterial invasion of the dentin is reviewed and the practice of removing all stain challenged. Article by Hien Ngo elsewhere in this issue presents practical clinical guidelines on how to do minimally invasive dentistry by taking advantage of bioactive restorative materials. In this article research showing internal remineralization underneath conventional glass ionomer suggests that this material constitutes a good method of treating the caries lesion chemically at the time of restoration. Article by Wang and Lussi elsewhere in this issue discusses the increasing problem of dental erosion (loss of tooth mineral from the surface due to acid sources other than bacteria). In contrast to caries disease, where the initial acid attack affects the enamel subsurface, in dental erosion stronger nonbacterial acids affect the surface layer directly.

SUMMARY

To conclude, there have been many exciting advances in our understanding of the caries process that should be changing the way we practice dentistry on a daily basis. This issue of *Dental Clinics of North America* helps to review and address these changes and the rationale behind them, as well as provide practical recommendations for clinical practice. There is a need to help bridge the gap between existing and newly developing evidence and routine practice, to improve the continuing dissemination of new information, and to enhance communication between dental research and the practice of dentistry in order to accelerate the implementation of validated approaches for the diagnosis and management of dental caries.[30] We have the responsibility as dental clinicians, researchers, and educators to use the best available evidence in the detection, assessment, management, and monitoring of caries lesions. How we choose to communicate and the nomenclature we use may greatly enhance or disrupt this process.

GLOSSARY
Dental Caries and Other Conditions that Also Result in Loss of Minerals from the Tooth

Dental caries
Is the localized destruction of susceptible dental hard tissue by acidic by-products from bacterial fermentation of dietary carbohydrates.[11] Thus, it is a bacterial driven, generally chronic, site-specific, multifactorial, dynamic disease process that results from the imbalance in the physiologic equilibrium between the tooth mineral and the plaque fluid; that is, when the pH drop results in net mineral loss over time.[31] The infectious disease process can be arrested at any point in time.

Dental fluorosis
Dental fluorosis is a hypomineralization of the dental enamel caused by excessive ingestion of fluoride during the transition and early maturation stages of enamel

development (eg, 15–30 months for central incisors). It is one of a variety of causes of defective enamel.[32]

Dental erosion
The clinical term dental erosion is used to describe the physical result of a pathologic, chronic, localized, loss of dental hard tissue chemically etched away from the tooth surface by acid and/or chelation without bacterial involvement. The acids responsible for erosion are not products of the intraoral flora; they stem from dietary, occupational, or intrinsic (eg, stomach acid associated with vomiting or gastroesophageal reflux) sources.[33,34]

Erosion, abrasion, and attrition are increasingly being termed "Tooth Wear." For example, the mechanisms of abrasion, erosion, and abfraction have been identified as causative agents of hard tissue loss at the cementoenamel junction (CEJ) of teeth. The etiology of these lesions appears to be multifactorial, with the association of patient factors being responsible for the various degrees of tooth wear.[35]

Abrasion
Abrasion is the pathologic wearing away of dental hard tissue through abnormal mechanical processes involving foreign objects or substances repeatedly introduced in the mouth and contacting the teeth.[33]

Demastication
Demastication describes the wearing away of tooth substance during the mastication of food with the bolus intervening between opposing teeth. Wear is then influenced by the abrasiveness of the individual food.[33]

Attrition
Attrition is the physiologic wearing away of dental hard tissue as a result of tooth-to-tooth contact, with no foreign substance intervening. Such contact occurs when grinding the teeth, for example, during swallowing and speech, and the resulting wear involves the occlusal and incisal surfaces of teeth.[33]

Abfraction
Abfraction is a wedge-shaped defect at the CEJ of a tooth caused by eccentrically applied occlusal forces leading to tooth flexure, which results in microfracture of enamel and dentine.[33]

The Caries Process and the Caries Lesion: Severity Stages, Activity

Caries process
The caries process is the dynamic sequence of biofilm-tooth interactions that can occur over time on and within a tooth surface.[11] This process involves a shift in the balance between protective factors (that aid in *remineralization*) and destructive factors (that aid in *demineralization*) in favor of demineralization of the tooth structure over time. The process can be *arrested* at any time.

Demineralization Demineralization is the loss of calcified material from the structure of the tooth. This chemical process can be biofilm mediated (ie, caries) or chemically mediated (ie, erosion) from exogenous or endogenous sources of acid (eg, from the diet, environment, or stomach).[11]

Remineralization Remineralization is the net gain of calcified material within the tooth structure, replacing that which was previously lost through demineralization.[11]

Arrest To stop a process; for example, efficient and frequent removal of the biofilm over a caries lesion that results in no further net loss of mineral from that previously active caries lesion.

Caries lesion/carious lesion
A caries/carious lesion is a detectable change in the tooth structure that results from the biofilm-tooth interactions occurring due to the disease caries.[11] It is the clinical manifestation (sign) of the caries process. "People have dental caries, teeth have caries lesions."[36]

Although attempts have been made in the literature to separate the term "caries lesion" from "carious lesion" (and in some cases to deprecate the term carious), the latter being used to refer in some instances to an "active" lesion, we find that applying those distinctions to everyday practice can be confusing and thus, we suggest that both terms can continue to be used interchangeably.

Caries lesion (pulpal) extent
A physical measurement/assessment of the net mineral loss in a pulpal direction. This can be graded, scaled, or measured as fractions of enamel and/or dentine thickness, in a pulpal direction, which have undergone net mineral loss.[11]

Caries lesion severity
This is the stage of lesion progression along the spectrum of net mineral loss, from the initial loss at a molecular level to total tissue destruction. This involves elements of both the extent of the lesion in a pulpal direction (ie, proximity to the dento-enamel junction and pulp) and the mineral loss in volume terms.[11] Noncavitated and cavitated lesions are, for example, two specific stages of lesion severity.

Noncavitated lesion
A noncavitated lesion is a caries/carious lesion whose surface appears macroscopically to be intact.[11] In other words, it is a caries lesion without visual evidence of cavitation. This lesion is still potentially reversible by chemical means, or arrestable by chemical or mechanical means. It is sometimes referred to as an *incipient lesion*, *initial lesion*, an *early lesion*, or *white-spot lesion* (even though color is very misleading as these lesions can be white, brown, and so forth).

White-spot lesion This is a noncavitated caries/carious lesion that has reached the stage where the net subsurface mineral loss has produced changes in the optical properties of enamel such that these are visibly detectable as a loss of translucency, resulting in a white appearance of the enamel surface.[11] However, it must be noted that although initial lesions appear as a white, opaque change to the naked eye, not all white-spot lesions are either initial (beginning lesions) or incipient, as they may be present for many years and may involve enamel and/or dentin.[31]

Brown-spot lesion A brown-spot lesion is a noncavitated caries/carious lesion that has reached the stage where the net subsurface mineral loss in conjunction with the acquisition of intrinsic or exogenous pigments has produced changes in the optical properties of enamel such that these are visibly detectable as a loss of translucency and a brown discoloration, resulting in a brown appearance of the enamel surface.[11]

Microcavity/microcavitation
A caries/carious lesion with a surface that has lost its original contour/integrity, without visually distinct cavity formation. This may take the form of localized "widening" of the

enamel fissure morphology beyond its original features, within an initial enamel lesion, and/or a very small cavity with no detectable dentine at the base.[11]

Cavity/cavitated lesion
A caries/carious lesion with a surface that is not macroscopically intact, with a distinct discontinuity or break in the surface integrity, as determined using optical or tactile means.[11]

"Caries free"
(Obsolete Term) This term has frequently been used when referring to assessments made (of either individuals or groups) even where the diagnostic threshold employed has been at the "dentine or worse" level, ignoring all grades of initial lesion that may also be present. The term should now be avoided and more precise terms used.[11]

"Active" caries
(Obsolete Term) This term was used to mean any lesion that had penetrated into dentine. The more modern definitions of "Activity" set out below (eg, active caries lesion) should now be used.[11]

Caries lesion activity (net progression toward demineralization)
The summation of the dynamics of the caries process resulting in the net loss, over time, of mineral from a caries lesion (ie, there is active lesion progression).[11]

Active caries lesion A caries lesion from which, over a specified period of time, there is net mineral loss, that is, the lesion is progressing.[11] Clinical observations to be taken into consideration for assessing caries lesion activity are based on a modification of the Nyvad and colleagues[37] caries lesion activity assessment criteria and the Ekstrand and colleagues[38] method. These criteria include visual appearance, tactile feeling, and potential for plaque accumulation: Lesion is likely active when surface of enamel is whitish/yellowish opaque and chalky (with loss of luster); feels rough when the tip of the probe is moved gently across the surface; lesion is in a plaque stagnation area, that is, pits and fissures, near the gingival and approximal surface below the contact point. In dentin, lesion is likely active when the dentin is soft or leathery on gently probing.[10,39] The term active caries should be avoided and replaced by active caries lesion.

Arrested or inactive caries lesion A lesion that is not undergoing net mineral loss; that is, the caries process in a specific lesion is no longer progressing.[11] It is a "scar" of past disease activity. Clinical observations to be taken into consideration for assessing caries lesion activity are based on a modification of the Nyvad and colleagues[37] caries lesion activity assessment criteria and include visual appearance, tactile feeling, and potential for plaque accumulation. Lesion is likely inactive when surface of enamel is whitish, brownish, or black; enamel may be shiny and feels hard and smooth when the tip of a probe is moved gently across the surface. For smooth surfaces, the caries lesion is typically located at some distance from the gingival margin. In dentin, the cavity may be shiny and feels hard on gently probing the dentin.[10,39]

Caries lesion regression
The net gain of calcified material to the structure of a caries lesion, replacing that which was previously lost through caries demineralization.[11]

Remineralized caries lesion A caries lesion that exhibits evidence of having undergone net mineral gain; that is, there is replacement of mineral previously lost due to the caries process.[11] In other words, this is a lesion that not only exhibits convincing evidence of lesion arrest but also one or more of other definite changes, including increased mineral concentration (remineralization): increased radiodensity, decreased size of white-spot lesions, increased hardness of the surface, and increased surface sheen compared with a previous matte surface texture.[40]

Hidden caries lesion
This is a term used to describe lesions in dentin that are missed on visual examination but are large enough and sufficiently demineralized to be detected radiographically. It should be noted that whether or not a lesion is actually hidden depends on how carefully the area has been cleaned and dried and whether criteria involving noncavitated stages of the caries disease process have been used or not.[31,41]

Classification of Lesions by Anatomic Location, Assumed Causality, and So Forth

Coronal primary caries lesion
Caries lesions produced by direct extension from an external surface in the coronal portion of a tooth.

Secondary caries, recurrent caries, or CARS—caries lesions associated with restorations and sealants
Caries lesions that occur at the margin of, or adjacent to, an existing filling.[42,43] These lesions have classically been described as occurring in two ways: an "outer lesion" and a "wall lesion." The chemical and histologic processes involved in "outer lesions" are the same as primary caries, and it has been suggested they occur as the result of a new, primary attack on the surface of the tooth adjacent to the filling. *Several researchers have suggested that secondary caries is quite likely to be primary caries adjacent to fillings.*[44,45] Thus, it has been recently suggested that these lesions be referred to as Caries lesions Associated with Restorations and Sealants (CARS).[10]

Residual caries lesion
Residual caries lesion is the part of a carious lesion left in a cavity preparation, either by oversight or purposely in an effort to avoid unnecessary dental pulp exposure, before a filling is placed.[31]

Root (Surface) caries lesion
Root caries lesions frequently are observed near the CEJ, although lesions can appear anywhere on the root surface. Root caries lesions appear as distinct, clearly demarcated circular or linear discolorations at the CEJ or wholly on the root surface.[10]

Pits & fissure caries lesions
Caries lesions that develop in the pit or fissure aspects of teeth.[10]

Approximal caries lesions
Caries lesions that develop in the mesial or distal surfaces of teeth.[10]

Free smooth surfaces caries lesions
Caries lesions that develop in the buccal or lingual surfaces of teeth.[10]

Rampant caries
This is a term sometimes used when multiple active caries lesions are occurring in the same patient. This usually also involves surfaces of teeth that normally do not experience caries (ie, mandibular incisors). Patients with "rampant caries" are sometimes classified by their assumed causality, for example, bottle or nursing caries, radiation caries.[31]

Early childhood caries (other terms that have been used in the literature: baby bottle syndrome, nursing bottle caries)
In accordance to the American Academy of Pediatric Dentistry,[46] Early Childhood Caries (ECC) is defined as the presence of one or more decayed (noncavitated or cavitated lesions), missing (due to caries), or filled tooth surfaces in any primary tooth in a child 71 months of age or younger. Furthermore, according to the AAPD,[46] any sign of smooth-surface caries in a child younger than 36 months of age indicates severe early childhood caries (S-ECC). From ages 3 through 5 years, one or more cavitated, missing (due to caries), or filled smooth surfaces in primary maxillary anterior teeth or a decayed, missing, or filled score of ≥ 4 (age 3), ≥ 5 (age 4), or ≥ 6 (age 5) surfaces constitutes S-ECC.[47]

Radiation caries
(Obsolete Term) Caries lesions of the cervical regions of the teeth, incisal edges, and cusp tips secondary to hyposalivation induced by radiation therapy to the head and neck.

Xerostomia (dry mouth) This term refers to a symptom and should be reserved for a patient's subjective feeling of oral dryness. The terms salivary hyposalivation and xerostomia are often incorrectly used interchangeably.[48]

Hyposalivation (hypoptylism) Hyposalivation is defined as a diminished secretion of saliva.[48] It may be associated with many factors alone or in combination, such as dehydration, radiation therapy for the salivary gland regions, anxiety, menopause, use of certain drugs, vitamin deficiency, inflammation or infection of the salivary glands, or various syndromes (eg, Sjögren).

Caries Detection, Assessment, Diagnosis, Monitoring, and Prognosis

Caries detection
Caries detection is a process involving the recognition (and/or recording), traditionally by optical or physical means, of changes in enamel and/or dentine and/or cementum, which are consistent with having been caused by the caries process.[11] In other words, it involves finding the signs (consequences) of the bacterial destruction of the dynamic caries process. Lesion detection, without assessment, is not practical or useful.[10]

Caries lesion assessment
Caries lesion assessment is the evaluation of the characteristics of a caries lesion once it has been detected. These characteristics may include optical, physical, chemical, or biochemical parameters, such as color, size, or surface integrity.[11]

Visual caries lesion assessment
Visual caries lesion assessment is the clinical evaluation of the characteristics of a caries lesion that relies on visual signs (change in color, cavitation), which represent manifestations of a relatively advanced caries process.

Caries disease diagnosis
Caries disease diagnosis is the human professional summation of all the signs and symptoms of disease to arrive at an identification of the past or present occurrence of the disease caries.[11] It involves the evaluation of host factors, saliva, diet, biofilm, and social, behavioral and psychological factors to determine the presence or not of the disease process.

Furthermore, *caries lesion diagnosis* is a process, which can be a stepwise procedure: detection of the lesion, followed by an assessment of the severity and extent of the lesion, as well as an assessment of the activity of the lesion.[49] To diagnose implies not only finding a lesion (detection) but, most importantly, to decide if it is active, progressing rapidly or slowly, or already arrested. Without this information a logical decision about treatment is impossible.[22]

"Watch"
(Obsolete Term) This is a term sometimes used to indicate early, white-spot lesions in either smooth or occlusal surfaces. The term is used to either indicate uncertainty regarding the state of activity of the lesion, or to indicate confusion uncertainty as to whether it is actually a caries lesion to begin with. As it is not a diagnostic term, it cannot lead to any management decision; the decision not to do anything or just "watch" should be eliminated from our choices of treatment. The term may have previously been used as a way to delay restorative intervention for sites that we were unsure about when we did not have many treatment options for these earlier stages of the disease. However, with the availability of better detection methods and noninvasive interventions, it is necessary to avoid using this term and make the best possible diagnostic call at any one point in time. Instead of "watching" over time, we should be "monitoring" the effect of our therapies and treatments on the lesions we are following.

Monitoring of a caries lesion
Monitoring is the assessment, over time, of one or more of the characteristics of a caries lesion to assess changes in that lesion.[11]

Caries lesion prognosis
Caries lesion prognosis is the likely future behavior of (or clinical outcome for) a specific caries lesion, over a specified time period, as assessed by a clinician, taking into account the summation of the multiple factors impacting on the possible progression, arrest, or regression of the lesion.[11]

Risk Assessment

Risk
Risk is defined as the probability that a harmful or unwanted event will occur.

Caries risk assessment
Caries risk assessment involves an analysis of the probability that there will be a change in the number, size, or activity of caries lesions.[21] The rationale of caries risk assessment is primarily to identify individuals with an increased risk for future disease development during a specified period of time. In addition, it would also be important to correctly identify those individuals with a risk of increased progression of the severity of the existing caries lesions.[50]

Unfortunately, there is no consensus in the literature concerning the use of the terms "risk factor" and "risk indicator." We have summarized available information in the definitions below.

Risk factor
Traditionally, a risk factor plays an essential role in the etiology of the disease, while a risk indicator is indirectly associated with the disease.[51] In other words, caries risk factors are the biologic reasons, or factors, that have caused or contributed to the disease, or will contribute to its future manifestation on the tooth.[15] A risk factor can, however, be strongly associated with a disease without being useful as a predictor. It is therefore suggested that the term "risk factor" should be exclusively used for variables established of value for prediction purposes in prospective studies.

The longitudinal design is thus required to evaluate whether a factor is a real risk factor, which means that it is present before the disease.[50] Therefore, a risk factor is an environmental, behavioral or biologic factor confirmed by temporal sequence, usually in longitudinal studies, which if present directly increases the probability of a disease occurring, and if absent or removed reduces the probability. Risk factors are part of the causal chain, or expose the host to the causal chain. Once disease occurs, removal of a risk factor may not result in cure.[52]

Risk indicator

Based on the previous discussion for the term risk factor, it follows that a risk indicator is a probable or putative risk factor, but the cross-sectional data on which it is based are weaker than the results of longitudinal studies.[52] In other words, the terms risk indicator/risk marker should be used for factors established in cross-sectional studies as being associated with the disease, in which correlations between various factors and the disease are investigated. A risk indicator, or combinations of several indicators, may very well be a risk factor if validated in prospective trials.[50]

However, please be aware that traditionally caries disease indicators have also been defined in a different manner in the literature. "They are clinical observations that tell about the past caries history and activity. They are indicators or clinical signs that there is disease present or that there has been recent disease. These indicators say nothing about what caused the disease or *how to treat it*. They simply describe a clinical observation that indicates the presence of disease. These are not pathological factors nor are they causative in any way. They are simply physical observations (holes, white spots, radiolucencies). The outcomes assessment described above, and prior literature, highlight that these disease indicators are strong indicators of the disease continuing unless therapeutic intervention follows."[15]

Caries protective factor

These are biologic or therapeutic factors or measures that can collectively offset the challenge presented by caries risk factors. The more severe the risk factors, the higher must be the protective factors to keep the patient in balance or to reverse the caries process.[15]

Prevention and Management

Caries prevention

"Preventive treatments" can be differentiated into 3 classic, sometimes overlapping, categories: primary prevention, secondary prevention, and tertiary prevention.[53]

Primary prevention

Includes those measures that prevent the development of the clinical signs of caries in the absence of disease, that is, prevent the initiation of the disease.

Secondary prevention

Centers on the prompt and efficacious treatment of disease at an early stage and includes measures that arrest and/or reverse the caries process after initiation of clinical signs.

Tertiary prevention

Involves measures that remove irreversibly damaged tooth tissue and replace it in such a way as to prevent further progress of the caries process.

(Note: some secondary and tertiary preventive options involve a "hybrid" interaction of nonoperative and operative procedures).

Continual monitoring and interventions based on risk factors, disease indicators, and protective factors to maintain oral health supports preventive treatment.

Caries Management by Risk Assessment is an evidence-based methodology where the clinician assesses risk factors for each individual patient—this is followed by diagnosis and prognosis of caries disease. Based on the evidence presented, the clinician then corrects the problems (by managing the risk factors) using specific treatment recommendations including behavioral, chemical, and minimally invasive procedures.[54]

Minimally invasive dentistry

Minimally invasive dentistry is supported by the emerging evidence and international consensus; it has an international focus, from for example the FDI World Dental Federation and others, and continues to be built on. The Minimal Intervention approach stresses a preventive philosophy, individualized risk assessments, accurate, early detection of lesions, and efforts to remineralize noncavitated lesions with the prompt provision of preventive care to minimize operative intervention. When operative intervention is unequivocally required, typically for a active cavitated lesion, the procedure used should be as minimally invasive as possible.[29]

What is not supported by the evidence or international consensus, but which is sometimes mislabeled as minimally invasive, is clinical activity in which small, early, and inactive/arrested lesions are sought out and prematurely or unnecessarily subjected to operative intervention.[11]

Minimally invasive dentistry (MID), minimal intervention (MI), and caries management by risk assessment (CAMBRA) are relatively new terms developed in response to scientific advances in the field. The terms are used interchangeably by some, and by others as a source of debate about which is the most proper term. For example, CAMBRA does not stop at prevention and chemical treatments; it includes evidence-based decisions on when, and how, to restore a tooth to minimize structural loss. In addition, MID and MI stand for much more than conservative cavity preparation. The term MI was endorsed by the FDI World Dental Federation in a 2002 policy statement[29] and is globally recognized. The terms CAMBRA and MID are in 100% agreement with the FDI statement on MI. Thus, the authors support the interchangeability of all 3 terms and recognize the importance of local preferences as well as global collaboration.[54]

ACKNOWLEDGMENTS

The authors would like to thank the thoughtful comments and review of Dr Spomenka Djordjevic, Dr Marcelle Nascimiento, and Shirley Gutkowski.

REFERENCES

1. Keene HJ. "History of dental caries in human populations: the First Million Years" animal models in cariology. In: Tanzer JM, editor. Proceedings, Animal Models in Cariology. Washington, DC: Information Retrieval Inc; 1981. p. 23–40.
2. Beltrán-Aguilar ED, Barker LK, Canto MT, et al. Surveillance for dental caries, dental sealants, tooth retention, edentulism, and enamel fluorosis—United States, 1988-1994 and 1999-2002. MMWR Surveill Summ 2005;54(No. SS–3):2–41.
3. Brown LJ, Wall MA, Lazar V. Trends in caries among adults 18-45 years old. J Am Dent Assoc 2002;133:827–34.

4. Dye BA, Tan S, Smith V, et al. Trends in oral health status; United States 1988-1994 and 1999-2004. National Center for Health Statistic. Vital Health Stat 11 2007;(248):1–92.
5. Sweeney PC, Nugent ZL, Pitts NB. Deprivation and dental caries status of 5 year old children in Scotland. Community Dent Oral Epidemiol 1999;27:152–9.
6. Lalloo R, Myburgh NG, Hobdell MH. Dental caries, socio-economic development and national oral health policies. Int Dent J 1999;49:196–202.
7. Reich E. Trends in caries and periodontal health epidemiology in Europe. Int Dent J 2001;51:392–8.
8. Pitts DB, Fejerskov O, von der Fehr FR. Caries epidemiology, with special emphasis on diagnostic standards. In: Fejerskov O, Kidd E, editors. Dental caries: the disease and its clinical management. Oxford (UK): Blackwell Publishing Ltd; 2003. p. 141–63.
9. Warren JA. Coming to terms with terminology. Oper Dent 1998;23(3):105–7.
10. International Caries Detection & Assessment System Coordinating Committee. The International Caries Detection And Assessment System (ICDAS II). Workshop sponsored by the NIDCR, the ADA, and the International Association For Dental Research. Available at: https://www.icdas.org. Accessed February, 2010. [Criteria Manual For The International Caries Detection And Assessment System (ICDAS II)].
11. Longbottom C, Huysmans MC, Pitts N, et al. Glossary of key terms. Monogr Oral Sci 2009;21:209–16.
12. Pitts NB, Stamm J. ICW-CCT statements. J Dent Res 2004;83(Special Issue C): 125–8.
13. Pitts NB. Modern concepts of caries measurement. J Dent Res 2004;83(Special Issue C):43–7.
14. Featherstone JD. The caries balance: the basis for caries management by risk assessment. Oral Health Prev Dent 2004;2(Suppl 1):259–64.
15. Featherstone JD, Domejean-Orliaguet S, Jenson L, et al. Caries risk assessment in practice for age 6 through adult. J Calif Dent Assoc 2007;35(10): 703–13.
16. Fontana M, Young D, Wolff M. Evidence based caries risk assessment and management. Dent Clin North Am 2009;53:149–61.
17. Pitts NB. Are we ready to move from operative to nonoperative/preventive treatment of dental caries in clinical practice? Caries Res 2004;38:294–304.
18. National Institutes of Health. Diagnosis and management of dental caries throughout life. Consensus Development Conference statement, March 26–28, 2001. J Dent Educ 2001;65:1162–8.
19. Bader JD, Shugars DA. Issues in the adoption of new methods of caries diagnosis. In: Stookey GK, editor. Early detection of dental caries. Indianapolis (IN): Indiana University School of Dentistry; 1996. p. 11–26.
20. Nyvad B. Diagnosis versus detection of caries. Caries Res 2004;38:192–8.
21. Fontana M, Zero D. Assessing patients' caries risk. J Am Dent Assoc 2006; 137(9):1231–40.
22. Kidd E. How clean must a cavity be before restoration? Caries Res 2004;38: 305–13.
23. Ismail AI. Visual and visuo-tactile detection of dental caries. J Dent Res 2004; 83(Special Issue C):56–66.
24. Ekstrand KR, Kuzmina I, Bjorndal L, et al. Relationship between external and histologic features of progressive stages of caries in the occlusal fossa. Caries Res 1995;29:243–50.

25. Ekstrand KR, Ricketts DN, Kidd EA. Reproducibility and accuracy of three methods for assessment of demineralization depth of the occlusal surface: an in vitro examination. Caries Res 1997;31:224–31.
26. Jablonski-Momeni A, Stachniss V, Ricketts DN, et al. Reproducibility and accuracy of the ICDAS-II for detection of occlusal caries in vitro. Caries Res 2008; 42:79–87.
27. Shoaib L, Deery C, Ricketts DNJ, et al. Validity and reproducibility of ICDAS II in primary teeth. Caries Res 2009;43:442–8.
28. Pitts NB. Introduction, how the detection, assessment, diagnosis and monitoring of caries integrate with personalized caries management. Monogr Oral Sci 2009; 21:1–14.
29. Tyas MJ, Anusavice KJ, Frencken JE, et al. Minimal intervention dentistry—a review. FDI Commission Project 1-97. Int Dent J 2000;50(1):1–12.
30. Fontana M, Zero D. Bridging the gap in caries management between research and practice through education: the Indiana University experience. J Dent Educ 2007;71(5):579–91.
31. Fejerskov O, Kidd EAM, Nyvad B, et al. Defining the disease: an introduction. In: Fejerskov O, Kidd E, editors. Dental caries: the disease and its clinical management. 2nd edition. Oxford (UK): Blakswell Munksgaard; 2008. p. 4–6.
32. Adair SM, Bowen WH, Burt BA, et al. Recommendations for using fluoride to prevent and control dental caries in the United States. Fluoride Recommendations Work Group. MMWR Recomm Rep 2001;50(Rr14):1–42.
33. Imfeld T. Dental erosion: definition, classification and links. Eur J Oral Sci 1996; 104:151–5.
34. Lussi A, Jaeggi T, Zero D. The role of diet in the aetiology of dental erosion. Caries Res 2004;38:34–44.
35. Bartlett DW, Shah P. A critical review of noncarious cervical (wear) lesions and the role of abfraction, erosion, and abrasion. J Dent Res 2006;85(4):306–12.
36. Steinberg S. Adding caries diagnosis to caries risk assessment: the next step in caries management by risk assessment (CAMBRA). Compend Contin Educ Dent 2009;30:522–35.
37. Nyvad B, Machiulskiene V, Baelum V. Reliability of a new caries diagnostic system differentiating between active and inactive caries lesions. Caries Res 1999;33(4):252–60.
38. Ekstrand KR, Ricketts DNJ, Kidd EAM, et al. Detection, diagnosing, monitoring and logical treatment of occlusal caries in relation to lesion activity and severity: an in vivo examination with histological validation. Caries Res 1998; 32:247–54.
39. Ekstrand KR, Zero DT, Martignon S, et al. Lesion activity assessment. Monogr Oral Sci 2009;21:63–90.
40. Anusavice KJ. Management of dental caries as a chronic infectious disease. J Dent Educ 1998;62(10):791–802.
41. Weerheijm KL, Gruythuysen RJ, Van Amerongen WE. Prevalence of hidden caries. ASDC J Dent Child 1992;59:409–12.
42. Mjör IA, Toffenetti F. Secondary caries: a literature review with case reports. Quintessence Int 2000;31:165–79.
43. Fédération Dentaire Internationale. A method of measuring occlusal traits. developed by the FDI commission on classification and statistics for oral conditions, working group 2 on dento-facial anomalies. Int Dent J 1973;23:530–7.
44. Kidd EAM, Beighton D. Prediction of secondary caries around tooth-colored restorations: a clinical and microbiological study. J Dent Res 1996;75:1942–6.

45. Ozer L. The relationship between gap size, microbial accumulation and the structural features of natural caries in extracted teeth with class II Amalgam restorations. Copenhagen (Denmark): University Of Copenhagen; 1997.
46. American Academy of Pediatric Dentistry. Policy on early childhood caries: classifications, consequences, and preventive strategies. Reference manual V30, N7. Available at: http://www.Aapd.Org/Media/Policies_Guidelines/P_Eccclassifications.Pdf. Accessed February, 2010.
47. Ismail AI, Sohn W. A systematic review of clinical diagnostic criteria of early childhood cries. J Public Health Dent 1999;59:171–91.
48. Navazesh M. How can oral health care providers determine if patients have dry mouth? J Am Dent Assoc 2003;134(5):613–8.
49. Ekstrand KR, Ricketts DN, Kidd EAM. Occlusal caries: pathology, diagnosis and logical management. Dent Update 2001;28:380–7.
50. Twetman S, Fontana M. Patient caries risk assessment. Monogr Oral Sci 2009;21:91–101.
51. Rothman KJ. Modern epidemiology. Boston: Little, Brown and Co; 1986.
52. Burt BA. Definitions of risk. J Dent Educ 2001;65(10):1007–8.
53. Longbottom C, Ekstrand K, Zero D. Traditional preventive treatment options. Monogr Oral Sci 2009;21:150–5.
54. Young D, Featherstone J, Roth JR, et al. Consensus statement caries management by risk assessment: implementation guidelines to support oral health. J Calif Dent Assoc 2007;35(11):799–805.

Microbiology of Dental Plaque Biofilms and Their Role in Oral Health and Caries

Philip D. Marsh, PhD[a,b,*]

KEYWORDS

- Dental plaque • Ecology • Biofilm • Dental caries
- pH • Interventions

Humans have an intimate and dynamic relationship with microorganisms. The human body is estimated to be composed of more than 10^{14} cells, of which only 10% are mammalian. The majority are the microorganisms that make up the resident microfloras that colonize all exposed surfaces of the body. The microfloras of the skin, mouth, and digestive and reproductive tracts are distinct from each other despite the frequent transfer of organisms between these sites; their characteristic composition is due to significant differences in the biologic and physical properties of each habitat.[1] These properties determine which microorganisms are able to colonize and which predominate or have only a minor role. This observation illustrates a key concept, namely, that the properties of the habitat are selective and dictate which organisms are able to colonize, grow, and be minor or major members of a microbial community.

The resident microfloras of the host not only reside passively at a site but also make an active contribution to the maintenance of health by (1) promoting the normal development of the immune system—some members of the resident microflora might also play a role in damping down deleterious immune responses,[2] and (2) excluding exogenous (and often pathogenic) microorganisms.[3] This latter process (colonization resistance) is due to the resident oral microflora being more competitive in terms of nutrient acquisition and attachment to oral receptors and by producing inhibitory molecules.

[a] Health Protection Agency, Centre for Emergency Preparedness & Response, Salisbury SP4 0JG, UK
[b] Department of Oral Biology, Leeds Dental Institute, Clarendon Way, Leeds LS2 9LU, UK
* Health Protection Agency, Centre for Emergency Preparedness & Response, Salisbury SP4 0JG, UK.
E-mail address: phil.marsh@hpa.org.uk

Dent Clin N Am 54 (2010) 441–454
doi:10.1016/j.cden.2010.03.002
0011-8532/10/$ – see front matter © 2010 Elsevier Inc. All rights reserved.

THE RESIDENT ORAL MICROFLORA

The mouth is similar to other habitats in the body in possessing a diverse but characteristic resident microbial community.[1,4] Bacteria are the most numerous group and, initially, they were characterized solely using cultural techniques. The recent application of molecular approaches that do not depend on prior cultivation for identification has provided deeper insights into the true richness of the resident oral microflora. It is now estimated that there are more than 700 different types of microbe that can be isolated from the mouth but that greater than 50% of these cannot currently be grown in pure culture in the laboratory.

The resident oral microorganisms obtain their nutrients primarily from endogenous sources, such as amino acids, proteins and glycoproteins in saliva, and gingival crevicular fluid; the metabolism of these substrates leads to only minor and slow changes to the local pH. Saliva also plays a major role in maintaining the oral pH at approximate neutrality, which is optimal for the growth of the majority of the microorganisms associated with oral health.[1,4] In contrast (discussed later), diet has a limited but generally deleterious impact on the balance of the resident oral microflora, mediated mainly by the rapid falls in pH in dental plaque.

The composition of the oral microflora varies significantly at distinct surfaces within the mouth (eg, tongue, buccal mucosa, and teeth), again due to differences in key environmental conditions.[1,4–6] This is despite the opportunity that bacteria have to colonize each site, and this observation further emphasizes the link that exists between the properties of the habitat and the organisms that are able to become established and predominate.

The resident microfloras on mucosal and dental surfaces in the mouth are examples of microbial biofilms. Biofilms are 3-D accumulations of interacting microorganisms attached to a surface, embedded in a matrix of extracellular polymers.[7–10] Research over the past decade has demonstrated that the properties of microbes attached to a surface as a biofilm are different from those expressed when the same organisms are grown under conventional conditions in a laboratory in liquid media. Of clinical relevance is the property that biofilms display increased tolerance to antimicrobial agents and to the host defenses.[11,12]

DENTAL PLAQUE BIOFILMS

The most diverse collections of oral microorganisms are found in the biofilms on teeth (dental plaque).[4–6] A small sample of dental plaque contains, on average, between 12 and 27 species.[5] These biofilms develop in a specific pattern. Within seconds of eruption, or after cleaning, tooth surfaces become coated with a conditioning film of molecules (biologically active proteins and glycoproteins) derived mainly from saliva (and also from gingival crevicular fluid and from the bacteria themselves).[13] Initially, only a few bacterial species are able to attach to this film, which is also termed, the *acquired pellicle*. Cells are held reversibly near to the surface by weak, long-range physicochemical forces. Molecules (adhesins) on these early bacterial colonizers, mainly streptococci (eg, *Streptococcus mitis* and *S oralis*) can bind to complementary receptors in the acquired pellicle to make the attachment irreversible[14] and then these pioneer species start to multiply. The metabolism of the early colonizers modifies the local environment, for example, by making it more anaerobic after their consumption of oxygen. As the biofilm develops, adhesins on the cell surface of more fastidious secondary colonizers, such as obligate anaerobes, bind to receptors on already attached bacteria by a process termed, *coadhesion* or *coaggregation*, and the composition of the biofilm becomes more diverse (*microbial succession*).[15] The attached bacteria produce extracellular polymers (the plaque matrix) that consolidate attachment of the biofilm. The matrix is more than a mere scaffold for the biofilm; the matrix can bind and retain molecules, including enzymes, and also retard the penetration of charged molecules into the biofilm.[16,17] Biofilms are spatially and functionally organized, and the heterogeneous conditions within the biofilm induce novel patterns of bacterial gene expression, while the close proximity of different species provides the opportunity for interactions.[18,19] Examples of these interactions include (1) the development of food chains (in which the end product of metabolism of one organism is used by secondary feeders) and metabolic cooperation among species to catabolize structurally complex host macromolecules; these interactions increase the metabolic efficiency of the microbial community; (2) cell-cell signaling, for example, by the secretion of small peptides to coordinate gene expression among cells of a similar species; (3) transfer of antibiotic resistance genes, and (4) antagonism by the production of inhibitory molecules, which may provide a competitive advantage to the producing organism or exclude undesirable microbes.[4]

Thus, dental plaque is a classic example of a biofilm and a microbial community, in which bacteria interact and the properties of the whole consortium are more than the sum of the constituent species. Additional information can be found in review articles that describe more fully the significance of dental plaque as a multispecies biofilm.[20–23]

The microbial composition of the biofilm varies at distinct sites on a tooth (fissures, approximal surfaces, and gingival crevice) and reflects the inherent differences in their anatomy and biology.[4,6] The normal microflora of fissures is sparse and the organisms present have a saccharolytic metabolism (ie, their energy is derived from sugar catabolism); the predominant bacteria are streptococci and there are few gram-negative or anaerobic organisms. In contrast, the gingival crevice has a more diverse microflora, including many gram-negative anaerobic and proteolytic species, whereas approximal surfaces have a microflora that is intermediate in composition.

Once established, the composition of the resident microflora at any site remains stable over time, unless there are marked changes to the habitat. This stability, termed *microbial homeostasis*, stems not from any metabolic indifference by the resident microflora but reflects a highly dynamic state in which the proportions of individual species are in balance due to the many interactions, both synergistic and antagonistic (described previously).[24] For example, long-term use of broad-spectrum antibiotics can suppress the resident bacterial oral microflora permitting overgrowth by previously minor populations of oral yeasts. This clinical observation demonstrates 2 principles. First, the resident oral microflora is responsive to environmental change and a major shift in local conditions can drive alterations in the composition and metabolic activity of the microflora that are deleterious to the health of the host, and, second, oral care practices should attempt to maintain plaque at levels compatible with health to retain the beneficial properties of the normal oral microflora.

DENTAL PLAQUE AND CARIES DISEASE

Many studies have been undertaken to determine the composition of biofilms from sites with caries lesions to try and identify the bacteria responsible for causing the demineralization. Interpretation of data from such studies is difficult because plaque-mediated diseases occur at sites with a pre-existing natural and diverse resident microflora. The anatomy of sites at risk for caries lesions means that there are intrinsic difficulties in taking discrete plaque samples. Traditional culture techniques have generally been applied to determine the bacterial composition of the plaque samples, but these approaches do not recover all of the microorganisms that are present, so potentially significant species could be underestimated or missed. Bifidobacteria are now being linked to caries disease etiology, but these bacteria have been difficult to isolate until recently when an effective selective medium for their detection was introduced.[25] There are wide intersubject variations in the composition of the plaque microflora from the same site, so that when data are averaged from many individuals, clear associations between bacteria and disease can be difficult to discern. In addition, the traits associated with cariogenicity (acid production, acid tolerance, and intracellular and extracellular polysaccharide production) are not restricted to a single species (discussed later).[26] Similarly, the consequence of acid production by cariogenic species can be ameliorated by the development of food chains with other plaque bacteria, such as Veillonella spp (which convert lactate to weaker acids), or due to alkali production (eg, ammonia generation from arginine or urea metabolism) by neighboring organisms.

Historical Perspective

Despite all these issues, progress has been made in determining the bacterial etiology of dental caries disease. In the late nineteenth century, Dr W.D. Miller put forward the "chemico-parasitic" theory of caries disease, in which he proposed that oral microorganisms can break down dietary carbohydrates to acids which demineralize enamel. Microbiology was in its infancy, however, and it was not possible to determine which bacteria were involved. In 1924, Clarke isolated streptococci from human caries lesions and named them S mutans. This finding was overlooked, however, for several decades, and it was not until the 1960s that further substantial progress was made when gnotobiotic animal studies were feasible and it could be shown categorically that (1) caries disease was a transmissible, (2) fermentable carbohydrates in the diet played a critical role, (3) oral streptococci (and other bacteria) from humans could cause caries lesions in rodents fed a high sugar diet, and (4) interventions, such as antibiotics targeted against these bacteria, prevented caries lesions. The most cariogenic species in these animal studies were what are now termed mutans streptococci, in particular S mutans and S sobrinus. These studies laid the foundation for epidemiologic studies in humans in which the prevalence and proportions of selected bacteria or the whole plaque microflora were compared at caries versus healthy surfaces. Detailed studies of the biochemistry and molecular biology of cariogenic bacteria have enabled the traits associated with cariogenicity to be identified. These include (1) the expression of high-affinity sugar transport systems for the uptake of fermentable carbohydrates and the rapid conversion of the transported sugars to acidic end products of metabolism (acidogenicity); (2) the ability to tolerate, grow, and continue to make acid in low-pH environments (aciduricity); (3) the synthesis of extracellular polymers (especially glucans and mutan) from sucrose to consolidate attachment; and (4) the production of intracellular polysaccharides during periods of excess carbohydrate availability; these storage compounds can be converted to acid during periods between meals when dietary sugars are not available.[27–29]

Human Epidemiologic Study Design

Two types of epidemiologic survey have been performed to determine the microbial etiology of caries disease. In cross-sectional surveys, predetermined caries-prone surfaces are sampled at a single time point, and the plaque microflora is related to the caries status of the site at that time. Large numbers of sites/people can be analyzed, and different age groups, tooth surfaces, diets, intervention strategies, and so forth can be compared. A major disadvantage of this study design, however, is that it cannot be determined for certain whether or not the species that are isolated from caries surfaces caused the decay or arose because of it; only associations can be derived from this study design. In contrast, longitudinal studies sample initially clinically sound sites at regular intervals over a set time period. Sites are selected on the basis of previous epidemiologic surveys, from which it can be predicted that a statistically relevant number of sites should suffer caries lesions within the time span of the study. The microflora can then be compared (1) before and after the diagnosis of disease and (2) between those sites that became diseased and those that remained healthy throughout the study, so that true cause-and-effect relationships can be established. These studies take longer to perform and are far more resource demanding (ie, expensive), so, for practical reasons, far fewer longitudinal studies have been performed.

Main Microbiologic Findings From Human Epidemiologic Studies

It is beyond the scope of this article to review the results from all of the studies performed on humans; more comprehensive reviews are recommended to readers.[27,28,30–32] Instead, data from some typical studies are highlighted to indicate the main trends.

Fissures are the most prone sites for caries lesions of the dentition, and the strongest correlation between the plaque levels of mutans streptococci and caries lesions has been found on these surfaces. For example, in a typical cross-sectional study, 71% of single fissures with open caries lesions in US children with rampant caries (and living in an area with a nonfluoridated water supply) had viable counts of mutans streptococci greater than 10% of the total cultivable plaque microflora, whereas 70% of fissures from similarly aged children who did not have visible caries lesions (but living in a community with water fluoridation) had no detectable mutans streptococci.[33] It was possible, however, to have a caries lesion in a fissure without detectable mutans streptococci as well as to find high levels of these bacteria in fissures that were diagnosed as being sound. In the same study, 65% of pooled plaque samples (approximal and occlusal surfaces of the 2 most posterior teeth) from children with rampant caries had counts of mutans streptococci greater than 10% of the plaque microflora whereas 40% of similar samples from children without any visible caries lesions had no detectable mutans streptococci. However, 16% of the pooled plaque samples from children with rampant caries had only low levels of mutans streptococci (<1% of the total plaque microflora).

In a longitudinal study of fissures in 52 US patients (aged 5 to 12 years) in which 4 examinations were performed at 6-month intervals, the proportions of mutans streptococci increased significantly at the time of lesion diagnosis.[34] The proportions of mutans streptococci reached almost 25% of the total fissure plaque in high caries active children at the time of diagnosis (compared with 7% and 10% at 12 and 6 months, respectively, before caries disease diagnosis). This trend was not observed in sound sites or in fissures that developed caries lesions but were in a low caries active group. Mutans streptococci were only minor components of plaque from 5 fissures that became carious, but these sites had high levels of lactobacilli, and these bacteria may have been responsible for the observed demineralization. A subsequent longitudinal study confirmed these findings and demonstrated an even stronger relationship between mutans streptococci and caries lesion initiation whereas lactobacilli, when present, were strongly associated with sites requiring restoration.[35]

A major prospective study of young Swiss children (aged 7–8 years) found that fissures and smooth surfaces of first permanent premolars that suffered demineralization without cavitation were heavily colonized with mutans streptococci (10^4–10^5

colony forming units/mL sample) at approximately 12 to 18 months before the clinical diagnosis of the lesion.[36] The proportions of mutans streptococci markedly increased 6 to 9 months before lesion detection, reaching 11% to 18% and 10% to 12% of the total streptococcal microflora of fissures and smooth surfaces, respectively. As with most studies on the microflora of caries disease, this study found some fissures with high levels of mutans streptococci but no discernible lesion, whereas other sites that had caries lesions had no detectable mutans streptococci at any time.

Challenges for studies of approximal surfaces lie with the difficulty in accurately detecting early lesions and with the fact that the biofilm is inevitably removed from the whole interproximal area, including that overlying sound as well as carious enamel. Early cross-sectional studies reported a positive correlation between elevated mutans streptococci levels and lesion development. A less clear-cut association was found in a large longitudinal study of 11- to 15-year-old UK children. At some sites, mutans streptococci could be found in high numbers before the radiographic detection of demineralization, whereas some lesions also developed in the apparent absence of these bacteria.[37] Mutans streptococci could also be present at some sites for prolonged periods in high numbers without any evidence of caries lesion development. The isolation frequency and proportions of mutans streptococci tended to increase after the first diagnosis of a lesion, especially in those that progressed deeper into the enamel, suggesting that the composition of the microflora might shift as the lesion progresses through the structure of the tooth. In a study in The Netherlands, mutans streptococci were isolated from 40% of sound sites and 86% of sites with caries lesions in Dutch army recruits aged 18 to 20 years, respectively.[38] In this study, S sobrinus (originally reported as S mutans serotype d) was recovered almost exclusively from recruits with caries lesions.

Rampant caries can occur in people who experience an exceptional change in the oral environment, such as those with markedly reduced salivary flow rates due to, for example, radiation therapy or medication. Longitudinal studies of patients undergoing radiation treatment showed large increases in the proportions of mutans streptococci and lactobacilli in plaque and saliva. These organisms also reach high levels in nursing bottle caries (early childhood caries), which occurs in young infants fed from bottles containing formula with a high concentration of fermentable carbohydrate.[27]

Collectively, the data from many surveys of various tooth surfaces, different patient age groups from many countries, populations with different dietary habits, and so forth, using conventional culture techniques, have shown a strong positive association between increased levels of mutans streptococci and the initiation of demineralization. This relationship is not absolute, however, and the majority of these epidemiologic studies report sites with mutans streptococci that are sound as well as surfaces that develop caries lesions in the apparent absence of mutans streptococci. In the latter samples, lactobacilli, bifidobacteria, Actinomyces spp, and low-pH non-mutans streptococci (streptococci that can generate acid and thrive at a low pH) have been implicated in caries lesion development.[25,39–41]

Contemporary studies have used molecular approaches to detect the predominant bacteria present in biofilms overlying lesions, without the bias introduced by the culturing of organisms on selective and nonselective agar plates. These studies generally have recovered a more diverse microflora, and novel taxa have been described.[42,43] One study confirmed the previously reported relationship of S sanguinis with sound enamel and S mutans and lactobacilli with caries lesions but additionally found Actinomyces gerencseriae and other Actinomyces spp implicated in caries lesion initiation and Bifidobacterium spp with advanced lesions.[44] Another study reported that 10% of subjects with rampant caries in the secondary dentition did not have detectable levels of *S mutans*.[45] In lesions where mutans streptococci could not be detected, there were high levels of lactobacilli, low pH–tolerating non-mutans streptococci, and *Bifidobacterium* spp. High levels of *Actinomyces* species and non-mutans streptococci were found in early (white spot) lesions, whereas mutans streptococci and lactobacilli, together with *Propionibacterium* and *Bifidobacterium* spp, dominated advanced lesions.[45] Often these detailed molecular studies have been performed on small numbers of samples, and more extensive investigations are awaited. A consistent trend is again emerging from these culture-independent studies in which, although mutans streptococci and lactobacilli are often associated with lesions, they are not always present, and a more diverse microflora is implicated.

Hypotheses to Explain the Role of Plaque Bacteria in the Etiology of Dental Caries Disease

From the start of the discipline of microbiology, it has been recognized that dental plaque biofilms have a diverse microflora. Therefore, it was a major advance when the specific plaque hypothesis was put forward.[46,47] This hypothesis proposed that only a few of the many species found in dental plaque biofilms are actively involved in disease. Thus, caries disease could be controlled by targeting preventative measures and interventions against these "specific" organisms, and the evidence at the time strongly implicated mutans streptococci as the main etiologic agent. Over time, as more studies identified sites where caries lesions developed in the absence of mutans streptococci, and there became a greater understanding of the metabolism of other members of the biofilm (eg, the role of bacteria that consumed acid or produced alkali), an alternative view on the role of plaque in caries lesion development was articulated. The nonspecific plaque hypothesis proposed that disease is the outcome of the overall activity of the total plaque microflora (as opposed to specific species), and, although often used in the context of periodontal diseases, the concept was also applied to caries disease.[48] The arguments about the merits of both hypotheses may seem to be about semantics, because plaque-mediated diseases are essentially polymicrobial infections in which only a few (perhaps specific) species are able to predominate. These hypotheses, however, also have implications for treatment strategies.[47] More general preventative approaches are warranted if a range of bacteria are involved whereas more specific interventions (targeted antimicrobials, vaccination) are justified if there is a more specific cause.

More recently, an alternative hypothesis was proposed (the ecological plaque hypothesis), which attempted to reconcile the key elements of the earlier 2 hypotheses and highlighted the critical role played by changes to the oral environment in predisposing an individual to caries disease.[49,50] Dental caries disease is viewed as a consequence of an imbalance in the resident microflora due to the enrichment within the microbial community of potentially more highly cariogenic bacteria due to frequent conditions of low pH in plaque biofilms, for example, as a result of a change to the diet or a reduction in saliva flow (**Fig. 1**). The application of more sensitive diagnostic methods has resulted in the frequent detection of mutans streptococci in plaque from healthy sites, albeit often in low numbers. These organisms are only weakly competitive with other oral bacteria at neutral pH and are present, therefore, as a small proportion of the total plaque community. In this situation, with a conventional diet, the levels of such potentially cariogenic bacteria are clinically insignificant, and the processes of de- and remineralization are in equilibrium. If the frequency of fermentable carbohydrate intake increases, then plaque spends more time below the critical pH for enamel demineralization (approximately pH 5.5). The effect of this on the microbial ecology of plaque is 2-fold. Conditions of low pH favor the proliferation of

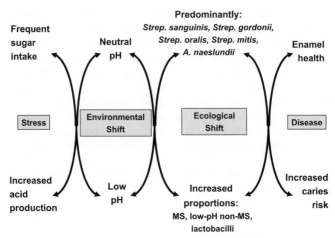

Fig. 1. The ecological plaque hypothesis. The diagram depicts the dynamic relationship that exists between the plaque biofilm and the local environment. When the frequency of intake of fermentable sugar increases, bacterial metabolism results in the biofilm spending more time at a low pH. An acidic pH inhibits the growth of many bacteria associated with enamel health while selecting for those bacteria with an acidogenic and acid-tolerating (aciduric) phenotype. Similar events occur if the flow of saliva is reduced. Under these conditions, demineralization is promoted, which increases the probability of a caries lesion developing. The caries process could be prevented not only by inhibiting the causative bacteria directly but also by interfering with the environmental changes that drive the deleterious shifts in the composition and metabolic activity of the biofilm. MS, mutans streptococci. (*Adapted from* Marsh PD. Microbial ecology of dental plaque and its significance in health and disease. Adv Dent Res 1994;8:263; with permission.)

acid-tolerating (and acidogenic) bacteria (including mutans streptococci, lactobacilli, and other bacteria with a similar phenotype) while tipping the balance toward demineralization (see **Fig. 1**). Greater numbers of bacteria, such as mutans streptococci and lactobacilli, in plaque result in more acid being produced at even faster rates, thereby enhancing demineralization and further disrupting the ecology of the biofilm. Other bacteria could also make acid under similar conditions, but at a slower rate, but could be responsible for the initial stages of demineralization or could cause lesions in the absence of more overt cariogenic species in a more susceptible host. If aciduric species were not present initially, then the repeated conditions of low pH coupled with the inhibition of competing organisms might increase the likelihood of successful colonization by mutans streptococci or lactobacilli. This sequence of events would account for the lack of total specificity in the microbial etiology of caries disease and explain the pattern of bacterial succession often reported during lesion progression.

The evidence for the ecological plaque hypothesis came from previously published clinical observations and from modeling studies performed in the laboratory in which mixed cultures of oral bacteria (representing those found in health and dental caries disease) were grown on mucin at neutral pH. Under these conditions, which mimic health, cariogenic species (S mutans and Lactobacillus rhamnosus) were uncompetitive with bacteria representative of enamel health and were less than 1% of the total microbial community. When the intake of dietary sugars was simulated by pulsing the cultures with glucose, there was little or no change in the proportions of the bacteria if the pH was maintained automatically at neutrality. If the pH was allowed to fall due to bacterial metabolism, however, there was a gradual and incremental shift in the balance of the microflora after each pulse, resulting in statistically significant increases in mutans streptococci and lactobacilli. After the final glucose pulse, these cariogenic species accounted for greater than 50% of the microflora, and the rate of acid production markedly increased.[51] Subsequent experiments showed that there was an inverse relationship between the terminal pH of the environment and the proportions of cariogenic bacteria whereas the converse was seen with bacteria associated with enamel health.[52] Inhibition of acid production by fluoride or xylitol reduced or prevented the selection of mutans streptococci.[53–55] These laboratory findings supported earlier clinical observations where increases in the proportions of mutans streptococci in plaque occurred when volunteers rinsed repeatedly with low-pH buffers.[56] Restriction of sucrose in the diet for as little as 3 weeks also led to a reduction in levels of mutans streptococci at sites with caries lesions and an increase in health-associated streptococci; this situation was rapidly reversed when a conventional sugar-containing diet was resumed.[57] These findings have implications for caries disease control and prevention; the data suggest that the selection of cariogenic bacteria could be prevented if the pH changes after sugar metabolism are reduced (discussed later).

Key features of the ecological plaque hypothesis are that (1) the selection of pathogenic bacteria is directly coupled to changes in the environment (see **Fig. 1**) and (2) diseases need not have a specific cause; any species with relevant traits could contribute to the disease process.[49,50] Thus, mutans streptococci are among the best adapted organisms to the cariogenic environment (high sugar/low pH) in having an acidogenic and aciduric phenotype, but such traits are not unique to these bacteria. Strains of other species possess some of these properties and, therefore, contribute to enamel demineralization. Considerable overlap also occurs in the expression of these cariogenic traits, so, for example, there is a range of acidogenicity and acid tolerance among strains of streptococci even within a species,[26] such that a weakly acidogenic strain of S mutans may not lower the pH as rapidly as a strain of S mitis with a higher glycolytic activity. A key element of the ecological plaque hypothesis is that disease can be prevented not only by targeting the putative pathogens directly (eg, by antimicrobial or antiadhesive strategies) but also by interfering with the selection pressures (high sugar/low pH) responsible for their enrichment.[49,50] In this way, clinicians become focused on treating the causes of a disease and not just the consequences of it.

A mixed-bacteria ecology approach has also been put forward[58]; in this, caries disease is dependent on the proportions and activity of acid- and alkali-producing bacteria in the biofilm. It was argued that the elimination of a specific organism, such as S mutans, would have little impact on caries disease, because other acidogenic bacteria would fill the vacated niche. The need for interventions that were targeted at mixtures of bacteria, and which could counter excessive acid production, was emphasized.[58]

An extension to the ecological plaque hypothesis has been proposed[59] in which bacterial adaptation occurs after transient exposure to conditions of low pH, resulting in the development of a more acidogenic/aciduric phenotype in normally weakly cariogenic bacteria.[60] In a dynamic stability stage, the biofilm is dominated by streptococci, such as S mitis and S oralis, and Actinomyces. Although these bacteria can produce acid from dietary sugars, the pH can be readily returned to neutrality and enamel can be remineralized. Under conditions of more frequent sugar metabolism, or if saliva flow is impaired, these streptococci and Actinomyces spp can adapt to conditions of low pH within the biofilm and develop a more enhanced acidogenic and aciduric phenotype. These changes in the biochemical activities of the microflora may tip the balance toward net mineral loss and thereby initiate lesion development (acidogenic stage) (**Fig. 2**). If the acidic conditions become prolonged and more common, then bacteria that are even more tolerant of low pH, such as mutans streptococci and lactobacilli, may out-compete other organisms within the biofilm and further accelerate the caries disease process (aciduric stage) and result in a less diverse (more extreme) microflora.[59]

Strategies that are consistent with the prevention of caries disease via the principles of the ecological plaque hypothesis, including the extended version, and which could augment conventional effective oral hygiene practices have been described[50] and include

Inhibition of plaque acid production (eg, by fluoride-containing products or other metabolic inhibitors, including xylitol). Fluoride improves enamel chemistry not only by enhancing remineralization and increasing resistance to acid but also by inhibiting several key bacterial enzymes, including some involved in glycolysis and in maintaining a favorable intracellular pH.[61] Xylitol cannot be metabolized to acid nor generate a low pH in plaque and may interfere with sugar transport in mutans streptococci. Inhibitors that reduce the pH fall in biofilms after sugar metabolism also prevent the establishment of environmental conditions in plaque that inhibit bacteria associated with sound enamel and favor growth of acid-tolerating cariogenic species.[53,54]

Avoidance between main meals of foods and drinks containing fermentable sugars or the promotion of consumption of foods/drinks that contain nonfermentable sugar substitutes, such as aspartame or polyols (eg, sorbitol and xylitol), thereby reducing repeated conditions of low pH in plaque.

Stimulation of saliva flow after main meals (eg, by sugar-free gum). Saliva introduces components of the host defenses, increases buffering capacity, removes

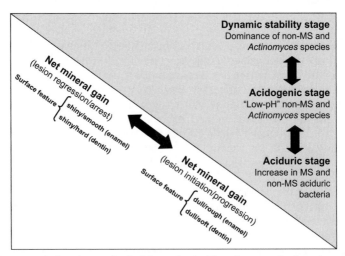

Fig. 2. The extended caries ecological hypothesis. The diagram depicts the relationship between acidogenic and aciduric (acid-tolerating) shifts in the composition of the dental biofilm microflora and changes in the mineral balance of the dental hard tissues. The sequence of ecological events is reversible and is reflected in the surface features of the dental hard tissues at any stage of lesion formation. MS, mutans streptococci. (*From* Takahashi N, Nyvad B. Caries ecology revisited: microbial dynamics and the caries process. Caries Res 2008;42:409; with permission.)

fermentable substrates, promotes remineralization, and returns the pH of plaque to resting levels more quickly.

Any other approach designed to maintain plaque pH at natural levels at approximate neutrality (eg, use of alkali-generating supplements, including arginine or urea).[50,59] Laboratory and clinical studies have provided proof that it is the low pH (generated from carbohydrate metabolism as well as other sources) that selects for mutans streptococci and other acidogenic/aciduric bacteria. Therefore, any approach that leads to the neutralization of these acids or prevents or reduces such a dramatic pH fall within the biofilm, helps in preventing catastrophic shifts in the plaque microflora and contributes to the maintenance of microbial homeostasis and, therefore, the beneficial properties of the normal microflora. More studies need to be done to evaluate products that could achieve this goal.

CONCLUDING REMARKS

The key to a more complete understanding of the role of microorganisms in dental caries disease depends on a paradigm shift away from concepts that have evolved from studies of classic medical infections with a simple and specific (eg, single species) etiology to an appreciation of ecological principles. The development of plaque-mediated disease at a site may be viewed as a breakdown of the homeostatic mechanisms that normally maintain a beneficial relationship between the resident oral microflora and the host. Microbial specificity in relation to caries disease needs to be considered in terms of microbial activity rather than simply the name of an organism. The traits (acid production, acid tolerance, and extracellular and intracellular polysaccharide production) associated with cariogenic bacteria are not specific to a particular species in the same way that toxin production by certain medical pathogens is diagnostic for that disease. These cariogenic traits are optimally expressed by mutans streptococci, but other bacteria also display these activities, to varying degrees, whereas there is also a spectrum of activity within the mutans streptococci.

When assessing treatment options, an appreciation of the ecology of the oral cavity enables enlightened clinicians to take a holistic approach and consider the nutrition, physiology, host defenses, and general well being of patients, because these affect the balance and activity of the resident oral microflora. After completion of a treatment plan, future episodes of disease inevitably occur unless the cause of any breakdown in homeostasis is recognized and remedied. For example, a side effect of many medications used by the elderly is a reduction in saliva flow. This has a deleterious impact on sugar clearance and buffering ability, thereby favoring the growth of acid-tolerating and potentially cariogenic bacteria. Identification of such critical control points in an evidence-based risk assessment program can lead to the selection of appropriate caries disease preventive strategies tailored to the needs of individual patients. In this way, clinicians not only treat the end result of the caries disease process but also attempt to identify and interfere with the factors that, if left unaltered, lead to more disease.

REFERENCES

1. Wilson M. Microbial inhabitants of humans. Their ecology and role in health and disease. Cambridge (UK): Cambridge University Press; 2005.
2. Cosseau C, Devine DA, Dullaghan E, et al. The commensal *Streptococcus salivarius* K12 downregulates the innate immune responses of human epithelial cells and promotes host-microbe homeostasis. Infect Immun 2008;76(9):4163–75.

3. Marsh PD. Role of the oral microflora in health. Microb Ecol Health Dis 2000;12: 130–7.

4. Marsh PD, Martin MV. Oral microbiology. 5th edition. Edinburgh (UK): Churchill Livingstone; 2009.

5. Aas JA, Paster BJ, Stokes LN, et al. Defining the normal bacterial flora of the oral cavity. J Clin Microbiol 2005;43(11):5721–32.

6. Papaioannou W, Gizani S, Haffajee AD, et al. The microbiota on different oral surfaces in healthy children. Oral Microbiol Immunol 2009;24(3):183–9.

7. Karatan E, Watnick P. Signals, regulatory networks, and materials that build and break bacterial biofilms. Microbiol Mol Biol Rev 2009;73(2):310–47.

8. Hall-Stoodley L, Stoodley P. Evolving concepts in biofilm infections. Cell Microbiol 2009;11(7):1034–43.

9. Hall-Stoodley L, Costerton JW, Stoodley P. Bacterial biofilms: from the natural environment to infectious diseases. Nat Rev Microbiol 2004;2(2):95–108.

10. Stoodley P, Sauer K, Davies DG, et al. Biofilms as complex differentiated communities. Annu Rev Microbiol 2002;56:187–209.

11. Stewart PS, Costerton JW. Antibiotic resistance of bacteria in biofilms. Lancet 2001;358:135–8.

12. Gilbert P, Maira-Litran T, McBain AJ, et al. The physiology and collective recalcitrance of microbial biofilm communities. Adv Microb Physiol 2002;46:203–55.

13. Hannig C, Hannig M, Attin T. Enzymes in the acquired enamel pellicle. Eur J Oral Sci 2005;113(1):2–13.

14. Whittaker CJ, Klier CM, Kolenbrander PE. Mechanisms of adhesion by oral bacteria. Annu Rev Microbiol 1996;50:513–52.

15. Kolenbrander PE, Palmer RJ Jr, Rickard AH, et al. Bacterial interactions and successions during plaque development. Periodontol 2000 2006;42:47–79.

16. Allison DG. The biofilm matrix. Biofouling 2003;19:139–50.

17. Vu B, Chen M, Crawford RJ, et al. Bacterial extracellular polysaccharides involved in biofilm formation. Molecules 2009;14(7):2535–54.

18. Kuramitsu HK, He X, Lux R, et al. Interspecies interactions within oral microbial communities. Microbiol Mol Biol Rev 2007;71(4):653–70.

19. Hojo K, Nagaoka S, Ohshima T, et al. Bacterial interactions in dental biofilm development. J Dent Res 2009;88(11):982–90.

20. Marsh PD. Dental plaque: biological significance of a biofilm and community lifestyle. J Clin Periodontol 2005;32:7–15.

21. Socransky SS, Haffajee AD. Dental biofilms: difficult therapeutic targets. Periodontol 2000 2002;28:12–55.

22. Filoche S, Wong L, Sissons CH. Oral biofilms: emerging concepts in microbial ecology. J Dent Res 2010;89(1):8–18.

23. Marsh PD. MoterA. Devine DA. Dental plaque biofilms: communities, conflict and control Periodontol 2000 2010, in press.

24. Marsh PD. Host defenses and microbial homeostasis: role of microbial interactions. J Dent Res 1989;68(Special issue):1567–75.

25. Mantzourani M, Gilbert SC, Sulong HN, et al. The isolation of bifidobacteria from occlusal caries lesions in children and adults. Caries Res 2009;43(4):308–13.

26. de Soet JJ, Nyvad B, Kilian M. Strain-related acid production by oral streptococci. Caries Res 2000;34:486–90.

27. Loesche WJ. Role of Streptococcus mutans in human dental decay. Microbiol Rev 1986;50:353–80.

28. Tanzer JM, Livingston J, Thompson AM. The microbiology of primary dental caries in humans. J Dent Educ 2001;65(10):1028–37.

29. Lemos JA, Abranches J, Burne RA. Responses of cariogenic streptococci to environmental stresses. Curr Issues Mol Biol 2005;7(1):95–107.
30. van Houte J. Role of micro-organisms in caries etiology. J Dent Res 1994;73(3): 672–81.
31. Marsh PD, Nyvad B. The oral microflora and biofilms on teeth. In: Fejerskov O, Kidd E, editors. Dental caries. The disease and its clinical management. 2nd edition. Oxford: Blackwell; 2008. p. 163–87.
32. Bowen WH. Do we need to be concerned about dental caries in the coming millennium? Crit Rev Oral Biol Med 2002;13(2):126–31.
33. Loesche WJ, Rowan J, Straffon LH, et al. Association of *Streptococcus mutans* with human dental decay. Infect Immun 1975;11(6):1252–60.
34. Loesche WJ, Straffon LH. Longitudinal investigation of the role of *Streptococcus mutans* in human fissure decay. Infect Immun 1979;26(2):498–507.
35. Loesche WJ, Eklund S, Earnest R, et al. Longitudinal investigation of bacteriology of human fissure decay: epidemiological studies in molars shortly after eruption. Infect Immun 1984;46(3):765–72.
36. Lang NP, Hotz PR, Gusberti FA, et al. Longitudinal clinical and microbiological study on the relationship between infection with *Streptococcus mutans* and the development of caries in humans. Oral Microbiol Immunol 1987;2(1):39–47.
37. Hardie JM, Thomson PL, South RJ, et al. A longitudinal epidemiological study on dental plaque and the development of dental caries—interim results after two years. J Dent Res 1977;56:C90–9.
38. Huis In 't Veld JH, van Palenstein Helderman WH, Dirks OB. *Streptococcus mutans* and dental caries in humans: a bacteriological and immunological study. Antonie van Leeuwenhoek 1979;45:25–33.
39. Sansone C, van Houte J, Joshipura K, et al. The association of mutans streptococci and non-mutans streptococci capable of acidogenesis at a low pH with dental caries on enamel and root surfaces. J Dent Res 1993;72(2):508–16.
40. Svensater G, Borgstrom M, Bowden GH, et al. The acid-tolerant microbiota associated with plaque from initial caries and healthy tooth surfaces. Caries Res 2003; 37(6):395–403.
41. van Ruyven FO, Lingstrom P, van Houte J, et al. Relationship among mutans streptococci, "low pH" bacteria, and iodophilic polysaccharide-producing bacteria in dental plaque and early enamel caries in humans. J Dent Res 2000; 79:778–84.
42. Chhour KL, Nadkarni MA, Byun R, et al. Molecular analysis of microbial diversity in advanced caries. J Clin Microbiol 2005;43(2):843–9.
43. Munson MA, Banerjee A, Watson TF, et al. Molecular analysis of the microflora associated with dental caries. J Clin Microbiol 2004;42(7):3023–9.
44. Becker MR, Paster BJ, Leys EJ, et al. Molecular analysis of bacterial species associated with childhood caries. J Clin Microbiol 2002;40(3):1001–9.
45. Aas JA, Griffen AL, Dardis SR, et al. Bacteria of dental caries in primary and permanent teeth in children and young adults. J Clin Microbiol 2008;46(4): 1407–17.
46. Loesche WJ. Chemotherapy of dental plaque infections. Oral Sci Rev 1976;9: 65–107.
47. Loesche WJ. Clinical and microbiological aspects of chemotherapeutic agents used according to the specific plaque hypothesis. J Dent Res 1979;58(12): 2404–12.
48. Theilade E. The non-specific theory in microbial etiology of inflammatory periodontal diseases. J Clin Periodontol 1986;13:905–11.

49. Marsh PD. Microbial ecology of dental plaque and its significance in health and disease. Adv Dent Res 1994;8(2):263–71.
50. Marsh PD. Are dental diseases examples of ecological catastrophes? Microbiology 2003;149:279–94.
51. Bradshaw DJ, McKee AS, Marsh PD. Effects of carbohydrate pulses and pH on population shifts within oral microbial communities *in vitro*. J Dent Res 1989;68: 1298–302.
52. Bradshaw DJ, Marsh PD. Analysis of pH-driven disruption of oral microbial communities *in vitro*. Caries Res 1998;32:456–62.
53. Bradshaw DJ, McKee AS, Marsh PD. Prevention of population shifts in oral microbial communities *in vitro* by low fluoride concentrations. J Dent Res 1990;69(2): 436–41.
54. Bradshaw DJ, Marsh PD. Effect of sugar alcohols on the composition and metabolism of a mixed culture of oral bacteria grown in a chemostat. Caries Res 1994; 28(4):251–6.
55. Bradshaw DJ, Marsh PD, Hodgson RJ, et al. Effects of glucose and fluoride on competition and metabolism within in vitro dental bacterial communities and biofilms. Caries Res 2002;36:81–6.
56. Svanberg M. *Streptococcus mutans* in plaque after mouth rinsing with buffers of varying pH values. Scand J Dent Res 1980;88:76–8.
57. de Stoppelaar JD, van Houte J, Backer-Dirks O. The effect of carbohydrate restriction on the presence of *Streptococcus mutans, Streptococcus sanguis* and iodophilic polysaccharide-producing bacteria in human dental plaque. Caries Res 1970;4:114–23.
58. Kleinberg I. A mixed-bacteria ecological approach to understanding the role of the oral bacteria in dental caries causation: an alternative to *Streptococcus mutans* and the specific-plaque hypothesis. Crit Rev Oral Biol Med 2002;13(2): 108–25.
59. Takahashi N, Nyvad B. Caries ecology revisited: microbial dynamics and the caries process. Caries Res 2008;42(6):409–18.
60. Takahashi N, Yamada T. Acid-induced acid tolerance and acidogenicity of non-mutans streptococci. Oral Microbiol Immunol 1999;14(1):43–8.
61. Marquis RE, Clock SA, Mota-Meira M. Fluoride and organic weak acids as modulators of microbial physiology. FEMS Microbiol Rev 2003;26(5):493–510.

The Caries Environment: Saliva, Pellicle, Diet, and Hard Tissue Ultrastructure

Anderson T. Hara, DDS, MS, PhD*, Domenick T. Zero, DDS, MS

KEYWORDS

- Caries environment • Salivary factors
- Dietary modifications • Tooth structure

An important starting place when discussing the caries environment is to accept that it is only the biofilm-covered tooth surfaces that have the potential to develop caries lesions. The multifaceted nature of the caries process makes it somewhat difficult to discuss any individual component in isolation of the other major etiologic factor, namely the dental biofilm. Thus, this article relates how saliva, the acquired pellicle, the diet, and the tooth structure itself interact and modify the pathogenicity of the dental biofilm, which is not necessarily pathogenic (see the article by Philip D. Marsh elsewhere in this issue for further exploration of this topic).

SALIVA

It is the saliva surrounding the tooth that creates the milieu that bathes the tooth surface and serves as the main vehicle for solubilizing and transporting potential harmful substances as well as protective factors to the biofilm-covered tooth surface. The saliva flow rate and composition are well recognized as important host factors that modify the caries process. Saliva's protective role is mediated by its ability to clear cariogenic food substances from the mouth; dilute, neutralize, and buffer organic acids formed by biofilm microorganisms; and reduce the demineralization rate and enhance remineralization by providing calcium, phosphate, and fluoride in the fluid phase of the biofilm in close association with the tooth surface. In that sense, aspects increasing the salivary flow rate, such as mechanical and chemical stimuli, are relevant modulating factors potentially increasing protection

Department of Preventive and Community Dentistry, Indiana University School of Dentistry, 415 Lansing Street, Indianapolis, IN 46202, USA
* Corresponding author.
E-mail address: ahara@iupui.edu

against caries lesion development. Mastication can stimulate the saliva output.[1] It has been suggested that stimulation of the mechanoreceptive neurons in the gingival tissues may result in a reflex secretion of saliva.[2] Chewing gum has proved to be an effective way to mechanically increase salivary flow. Clinical studies have been able to correlate sugarless gum use with lower levels of caries lesions.[3–8] Although no clear association has been observed with the presence of specific ingredients of the gum (ie, sugar substitutes such as sorbitol or xylitol), a rather evident benefit seems to be related to the mechanical stimulation of saliva by the chewing process.[8] Chemical stimulation from acidic food has been shown to significantly increase salivary flow.[9] Depending on the stimuli, different salivary glands may be affected leading to the variation in salivary flow and composition,[9] thus influencing the level of salivary protection.

Higher salivary flow allows for increased availability of organic and inorganic constituents of saliva. The inorganic constituents of interest are calcium (Ca^{2+}), phosphate (PO_4^-), fluoride (F^-), carbonic acid (H_2CO_3)/hydrogen carbonate (HCO_3^-), and di-hydrogenphosphate ($H_2PO_4^-$)/hydrogenphosphate (HPO_4^{2-}).[10,11] These ions are associated with the maintenance of the integrity of teeth by regulating the demineralization/remineralization processes and the buffer capacity of saliva.[12] Although the benefits of calcium phosphate and fluoride have been well established,[13] the influence of salivary buffer capacity in the prevention of caries is not well defined and has sometimes been questioned.[14–16] However, it has been reported that the concentration of hydrogen carbonate, the main buffer component of saliva, increases about 12 times from unstimulated to stimulated whole saliva.[17] Therefore, the salivary buffer capacity can be considered as a potential contributing factor in the reduction of enamel demineralization, although its effect may, sometimes, be overshadowed by several other caries risk factors such as oral hygiene, presence of cariogenic bacterial strains, sugar consumption, and fluoride.[18] Thicker biofilms that form in caries-prone tooth surfaces may limit the ability of saliva to exert its protective effect in combination with the interactions that occur between cariogenic bacteria and diet.

Increase of salivary flow has a direct impact on the clearance of sugar and acids from the tooth surface, which implicates the onset and progression of dental caries lesions. Once secreted into the mouth, saliva will form a thin film that interacts with substances present on the teeth and/or mucosa surfaces that will be ultimately removed from the oral cavity by swallowing.[19] The rate of oral clearance was shown to vary markedly at different locations in the mouth.[20,21] Oral clearance is slower for upper teeth compared with lower and for the buccal surfaces compared with lingual. The slowest clearance rate is on the buccal surface of the upper anterior teeth, whereas the fastest is on the lingual surfaces of lower anterior teeth. This can be explained by the proximity of those surfaces in relation to the submandibular and sublingual glands. More recently, the importance of the location of the parotid duct orifice was also shown to be important for the clearance rate of buccal surfaces of upper molars.[22]

If the increase of salivary flow benefits caries prevention, the loss of salivary function has shown to be detrimental and can be associated with the development of rampant caries lesions.[23,24] Salivary flow impairment can be related to aging[11,25,26] even though some other studies have not found this correlation.[27,28] It is well established that patients taking medication can also present decreased saliva output,[29] as well as those who have received radiation therapy for neck and head cancer.[30] Tests of the stimulated and unstimulated flow rate as well as of the buffer capacity of saliva may provide useful information about the susceptibility of an individual to dental caries. It is suggested that sialometric evaluations be carried at a fixed time point or in a limited time interval in the morning, avoiding intraindividual variations owing to the circadian cycle.[31]

The organic phase of saliva contains antimicrobial agents, such as secretory immunoglobulin A (IgA), lysozyme, lactoferrin, and peroxidases that may be related to caries.[32] Lysozyme can lead to bacteriolysis by disrupting bacterial cell walls. Lactoferrin binds iron, interfering with bacterial growth by both iron-dependent and -independent mechanisms. Lactoperoxidase can oxidize bacterial sulfhydryl groups, thus inhibiting glucose metabolism.[33] This peroxidase protects salivary glycoproteins from degradation by bacteria. Salivary IgA can react with *Streptococcus mutans;* consequently, it may have implications on the prevention of dental caries.[34,35] Studies have suggested that saliva of caries-free patients contains higher levels of IgA antibody against many *S mutans* epitopes than the saliva of caries-susceptible patients[35–37]; however, the strength of these relationships may not be adequate to have clinically useful predictive value.

The organic phase of saliva is also constituted by proteins that may regulate the demineralization and remineralization processes involved in caries development and arrest. Statherins,[38–40] proline-rich proteins (PRPs),[38,41] histatins,[42] and cystatins[43] have shown high affinity to enamel surfaces and are potentially involved with the maintenance of tooth integrity by supporting a suitable calcium phosphate environment. Thus, it is suggested that those salivary proteins can provide protection against demineralization. Up to this date, the literature is scarce showing how this interaction occurs in clinically relevant conditions and what would be the net result in terms of demineralization and remineralization of the dental structures. Mandel and colleagues[44] and Mandel and Bennick[45] could not observe differences between caries-active and caries-resistant individuals when analyzing parotid saliva proteins and acidic PRPs, respectively. Conversely, Balekjian and colleagues[46] found that rampant caries was associated with the reduction in the proportion of basic proteins and increase in amylase. Vitorino and colleagues,[47] using mass spectrometry approaches, showed a strong correlation between presence of phosphoproteins (PRP1, PRP3, histatin 1, and statherin) and absence of caries, suggesting that large amounts of phosphoproteins could contribute to more effective remineralization processes. More recently, Rudney and colleagues[48] similarly identified not only statherin but also cystatin s-(AA1-8) variant as predictors of occlusal caries. Higher levels of these proteins seemed to be associated with higher rates of remineralization. Although the above-mentioned studies may suggest some relevance of the salivary proteins in the maintenance of tooth surface integrity, results are still inconclusive. Dodds and colleagues[11] have suggested that not only the proteins but also their biologic activity are relevant for the development of caries lesions. In addition, limitations on the experimental design may interfere with the results.[11] More research is needed to verify how those, and potentially other salivary proteins, can modify the caries process.

Considering the importance of saliva in the caries process, attempts have been made to evaluate its properties and composition and use them to predict the development of caries. For instance, clinical tests and tool kits have been developed to evaluate the salivary flow (unstimulated and stimulated) and the inorganic phase of saliva, including its pH, buffer capacity, and Ca^{2+}, PO_4^{3-}, and F^- ion concentrations. Similarly, it has been suggested that salivary proteins could be used as key biomarkers for several systemic diseases, including dental caries.[49–51] The collection of information on the salivary factors may be of great help in determining the individual risk for caries development, but additional validation is required.

ACQUIRED PELLICLE

The acquired pellicle is an acellular, bacteria-free organic film that is deposited on teeth, occupying a critical position between the enamel surface and dental biofilm. The pellicle is formed mainly by the salivary glycoproteins and proteins from different sources, including saliva, bacterial components or products, gingival crevicular fluid, blood, food, and enamel fluid.[52] These select organic components have a high affinity for the enamel surface and rapidly adsorb to a clean (after tooth brushing with dentifrice, chemical dissolution, or prophylaxis) enamel surface. The pellicle formation process appears to involve a 2-step process.[53] Initially, there is adsorption of discrete proteins to the hydrophobic regions of the tooth by electrostatic interactions, leaving hydrophobic parts of the protein molecules exposed at the surface. Following, protein aggregates or micellelike structures may adsorb to uncovered sites on the tooth surface and also interact with the initially formed hydrophobic protein layer.[53,54] This specific adsorption pattern seems to be responsible for the globular morphology of the acquired pellicle.[55,56]

This organic layer becomes detectable on dental surfaces after a few minutes of exposure to the oral environment.[53,57] Biologic, ie, enzymatic, activity is also detectable on early stages of pellicle formation.[58,59] It is suggested that it grows until reaching equilibrium between protein adsorption and de-sorption within 2 hours.[60] Even if the pellicle may reach its full thickness in 2 hours, there is a continuing maturation process, which modifies the pellicle characteristics as a diffusion barrier to ionic conductivity on the enamel surface.[61–64] In in vitro conditions, this maturation process was suggested to take at least 4 days, whereas about 18 hours was needed in in vivo conditions. It seems that enzymes, possibly transglutaminase,[65,66] may account for this difference.[60] Transglutaminase is continuously resupplied in the mouth but, because of its short half-life, rapidly loses its activity in vitro. Therefore, enzyme activity promotes a structural remodeling of the acquired pellicle during the maturation process,[59] which seems to be important for stabilizing and creating a more acid-resistant pellicle.[60] Extraoral factors may also modify pellicle formation. The regular use of abrasive toothpastes, whitening products, intake of acidic foods and beverages, and the frequent abrasion of teeth during professional cleaning inhibit pellicle formation and maturation. This may increase the susceptibility of enamel to dental erosion[67] and potentially modify the caries susceptibility of a tooth surface.

Similar to saliva, the acquired enamel pellicle is constituted of proteins such as albumin, mucin, acidic PRPs, and cystatins that have shown to be important contributors to the protection of enamel tissues from acid-induced demineralization.[61,68–70] The acquired pellicle can act not only as a physical barrier preventing acid diffusion,[57] but also as a reservoir of remineralizing electrolytes (Ca^{2+}, PO_4^{3-}, and F^-).[59] Recent developments of sensitive proteomic methodologies have opened new avenues for the characterization of very low abundance biologic samples. Using this proteomic technology, more than 130 different proteins have been identified in the dental pellicle[71,72]; however, there is no clear understanding of their roles in dental caries development. It is known that those proteins can modulate the mineral homeostasis of tooth surfaces and the attachment of the bacteria that constitute the oral biofilm.

The thickness of the acquired enamel pellicle is reported to be between 0.1 and 1.0 µm. Besides acid demineralization protection, the pellicle serves as a lubricant between teeth and soft tissues and other structures, allowing free movement. More importantly for the current topic, the pellicle also provides a base for the subsequent development of dental biofilm. Early colonizing bacteria derived from the saliva passively adhere to this pellicle. In this process, statherin and PRPs seem to have active roles, as they have anchoring receptors that allow microorganisms to attach firmly to their surfaces by electrostatic, hydrophobic ionic, and van der Waals forces. The maturation of the dental biofilm as well as its pathogenicity is further described in the article by Philip D. Marsh elsewhere in this issue.

DIET

Dental caries has long been associated with the frequency of fermentable carbohydrate intake. Changes in dietary patterns and the increase in the use of fluoride has modified this relationship, as discussed later; however, from an etiology basis, diet still remains the main driver of the caries process. In that aspect, considerations on the retentiveness of the food, the presence of protective factors in foods (calcium, phosphate, and fluoride), and the type of carbohydrate are still important. Relevant carbohydrates can be divided into complex and simple. Complex carbohydrates (starches) are considered less cariogenic because starches are not readily soluble in oral fluids and have a low diffusion rate in biofilm. They also must be broken down to maltose by salivary amylase before biofilm bacteria can metabolize them; however, most starch is cleared from the mouth before it can be broken down. Simple sugars (sucrose, glucose, fructose) are more cariogenic, with sucrose being possibly the most; therefore, it has been implicated as an important determinant of dental caries disease.[73,74]

Sucrose represents the main source of sugar in the diet. In studies in rats, using an experimental caries model, sucrose was shown to be more cariogenic than other dietary sugars such as glucose, fructose, and lactose. This cariogenic effect appears to be strain-specific, and is also influenced by the type of animal model and class of caries.[75] The cariogenic properties of sucrose may be explained by 2 main processes. First, sucrose is freely diffusible in dental plaque and readily metabolized by oral bacteria, leading to the production of organic acids in sufficient concentration to lower the pH of dental plaque enough to allow enamel demineralization to occur. Second, sucrose is involved in the synthesis of soluble and insoluble extracellular glucan. The enzymes responsible for the synthesis of extracellular glucans and fructans (glucosyltransferases and fructosyltransferases, respectively) have a high affinity for sucrose. Although the first property is shared among simple sugars, the second is specifically related to sucrose only.

The synthesis of extracellular polysaccharides can favor the accumulation of *S mutans* and other cariogenic bacteria in dental biofilm.[76,77] This unique property of sucrose has been shown in previous studies using an intraoral caries model, where markedly enhanced demineralization was associated with *S mutans* test plaques prepared from sucrose-containing cultures compared with glucose-grown plaques.[78] This was attributed to an alteration of the diffusion properties of plaque owing to the presence of water-insoluble extracellular matrix material (glucan) synthesized from sucrose.[79–81] The extracellular matrix permits greater penetration of dietary carbohydrates into the deeper layer of dental biofilm adjacent to the tooth surface, which from a caries lesion point of view is the only layer that counts.

It is important to keep in mind that the relationship of diet with caries disease has changed.[82] All historical and epidemiologic evidence before 1970 clearly associated the availability of sugar and refined carbohydrates with increased caries disease prevalence.[83] Caries disease increased in severity as the standard of living and nutrition improved. From the early 1970s until the most recent (1999–2004) US National Health and Nutrition Examination Survey,[84] a change has been observed in that there has been a reduction in the caries prevalence in adolescents (age 12 to 19), adults (age 20 to 64), and seniors (age 65 and older). There was, however, a small but significant increase in caries in the primary teeth of children (age 2–11). Although no clear change has been observed in total sugar consumption over the past 30 years, there has been a change in the form of sugar use, with reduction of sucrose and increase of fructose use, mainly in the form of high-fructose corn syrup.[85] Although the reduction in caries prevalence has been generally attributed to topical effects of fluoride, the reduction in sucrose consumption and replacement with other simple sugars may also be a contributing factor.

Individual guidance on dietary changes should be provided by dental care practitioners. This includes the assessment of the patient's dietary habits with analyses of the sugar exposure patterns and type of foods. This information can be obtained through the use of dietary diaries and also by recall interviews. Diet counseling should focus not only on reducing the exposures to sugar but also on providing recommendations of healthier alternatives.[86]

TEETH

Host factors involved in the caries process are the location, morphology, composition, ultrastructure, and posteruptive age of the tooth. Enamel is composed mostly of mineral in the form of hydroxyapatite (HAp), chemically represented by $Ca_{10}(PO_4)_2(OH)_2$. However, enamel should not be considered as pure hydroxyapatite,[87] because it also contains organic components and some of the HAp ions can be generally substituted, affecting the stability and acid solubility of the crystals composing enamel. Depending on the substitutions involved, the final mineral composing the human enamel and dentin can be more or less soluble to acids than the pure form of HAp.[88] Therefore, theoretically, if one could decrease the acid solubility of enamel, this would decrease the caries susceptibility of a tooth. However, studies have shown that even pure fluorapatite, which is the least acid-soluble calcium phosphate species, will demineralize in the presence of a strong acid challenge.[89]

Ultrastructurally, the acid solubility of a tooth and thus its caries resistance can be affected by the crystal size and shape, and the proximity of the crystals. The mineral composition differences will determine the stability of the crystals forming the structure of enamel, affecting its solubility. The more stable the crystals, the less soluble they will be. Fluorapatite (substitution of OH^- by F^- ions) is a highly stable crystalline form, even more than hydroxyapatite, which explains its lower solubility. Substitution of PO_4^{3-} ions by carbonate, on the other hand, renders enamel less stable and consequently more susceptible to demineralization. Carbonate is present in relatively high levels when teeth erupt.[90] Other elements present in the physiologic fluid, during enamel development, can also be incorporated into enamel.[91] More than 40 trace elements have been identified in enamel. These trace elements can be incorporated into enamel in various ways: ion exchange in the hydration shell, which is the layer of water adjacent to the crystal; direct absorption on the surface of the crystal; and substitution with components of the crystal of similar size and charge (ie, F^- for OH^-, Sr^{2+} for Ca^{2+}, and CO_3^{2-} for PO_4^{3-}). Different geographic areas are known to have different levels of trace elements in the soil and drinking water, which are reflected in the composition of enamel.[92] However, differences in the trace element composition of teeth are considered to be of only minor overall importance to the caries process. Even fluoride levels in teeth are not strongly correlated with caries disease experience.

Enamel is composed of long, thin crystallites (<40 nm in diameter) bundled together to form enamel rods or prisms (<4 μm in diameter) surrounded by an organic matrix forming the prism sheath.[93] The prisms run from the dentin to outer enamel surface.

Larger, more uniform crystals have less specific surface area and thus are less reactive (less acid soluble).[94] Enamel has the properties of a microporous material. The water-filled spaces between the crystals serve as diffusion channels where acids can diffuse to attack the crystals. The closer the crystals are packed, the less space there is for water diffusion, thus reducing enamel solubility.

Another important consideration is the dynamic environment created by the interaction between the enamel surface and the dental biofilm. Following eruption in the oral cavity, the enamel surface undergoes a maturation process. The caries process involves repeated episodes of demineralization and remineralization, which over time renders enamel more resistant to subsequent acid challenge.[95] Therefore, caries lesion susceptibility of the enamel surface is greatest immediately after eruption and tends to decrease with age,[96,97] as the enamel surfaces continuously react with the oral environment. Biofilm acids first attack the more soluble carbonate-rich apatite leaving the less soluble mineral phase. Over time the partially demineralized enamel is remineralized with apatite lower in carbonate and higher in fluoride that is less acid soluble.[90] Additionally, organic material is deposited into voids created by the demineralization, which is thought to have a protective role.[98] The mechanism of action of fluoride is closely tied to its ability to enhance remineralization and thus accelerate the posteruptive maturation of the tooth structure.[99]

Enamel is the most at-risk surface for caries lesions and thus has received the most attention. More recently, dentin has also been considered. Because teeth are being kept in the mouth longer, exposure of coronal dentin as well as of root dentin is becoming clinically common as a result of tooth wear and gingival recession, respectively. Dentin is relatively more soluble than enamel, presenting a critical pH value of about 6.2 to 6.7.[100,101] Therefore, critical differences should be expected regarding caries lesion susceptibility and progress.

Changes in the mineral and fluoride content of enamel and dentin may also influence caries progress. Previous loss of the enamel surface by caries disease or erosive-abrasive processes may increase the susceptibility to demineralization, as the surface layer is known to have a higher content of fluoride and to be more acid resistant. Conversely, remineralized enamel surfaces in the presence of fluoride may present acid-resistant crystals of fluoridated apatite,[95] reducing further demineralization episodes. Remineralized and sclerotic dentin have been reported as result of caries lesions and injuries to the pulp, respectively, and should also have different susceptibilities to demineralization. Studies have shown that these substrates may be less prone to demineralization[102,103] and consequently to caries progress. Exposure of saliva to dietary products rich in Ca and PO_4 and to fluoride has shown to be effective in remineralization of the demineralized enamel, once the cariogenic biofilm is neutralized or removed from the tooth surface and the pH rises above the critical level for dental demineralization.

Recently, given the increasing attention dispensed to esthetic dental procedures, dental bleaching has been investigated with respect to the possible detrimental side effects on enamel and dentin. It has been shown that some hydrogen peroxide–based gels may influence enamel surface morphology[104,105] and softening,[104,106,107] suggesting, thus, some influence on increasing the susceptibility of tooth to demineralization. These changes are thought to be related to specific experimental conditions adopted or to the properties of the products. In some tests, neither artificial nor human saliva was used to allow the bleached teeth to remineralize, simulating the clinical conditions. Similar studies considering remineralization by saliva during and after the bleaching treatment have showed no damage to the enamel and dentin surfaces.[108–110] The concentration of hydrogen peroxide and also the pH of the bleaching agent[111,112] should be considered. Some bleaching agents have a high content of hydrogen peroxide and a low pH value, under the critical pH of enamel and dentin. However, the use of bleaching agents with lower content of hydrogen peroxide and neutral pH has not been reported to be harmful to the tooth structure.

SUMMARY

The caries process can be understood in very simple terms as being the result of acids generated by the dental biofilm from dietary fermentable carbohydrates causing demineralization of tooth mineral and ultimately leading to a caries lesion. However, the complex and dynamic environment created by interactions among dental biofilm, saliva, acquired pellicle, diet, and hard tissue itself must be taken into account to fully understand the caries disease process.

REFERENCES

1. Yeh CK, Johnson DA, Dodds MW, et al. Association of salivary flow rates with maximal bite force. J Dent Res 2000;79(8):1560–5.
2. Scott BJ, Bajaj J, Linden RW. The contribution of mechanoreceptive neurones in the gingival tissues to the masticatory-parotid salivary reflex in man. J Oral Rehabil 1999;26(10):791–7.
3. Möller IJ, Poulsen S. The effect of sorbitol-containing chewing gum on the incidence of dental caries; plaque and gingivitis in Danish schoolchildren. Community Dent Oral Epidemiol 1973;1(2):58–67.
4. Glass RL. A two-year clinical trial of sorbitol chewing gum. Caries Res 1983; 17(4):365–8.
5. Mäkinen KK, Bennett CA, Hujoel PP, et al. Xylitol chewing gums and caries rates: a 40-month cohort study. J Dent Res 1995;74(12):1904–13.
6. Beiswanger BB, Boneta AE, Mau MS, et al. The effect of chewing sugar-free gum after meals on clinical caries incidence. J Am Dent Assoc 1998;129(11): 1623–6.
7. Szöke J, Bánóczy J, Proskin HM. Effect of after-meal sucrose-free gum-chewing on clinical caries. J Dent Res 2001;80(8):1725–9.
8. Machiulskiene V, Nyvad B, Baelum V. Caries preventive effect of sugar-substituted chewing gum. Community Dent Oral Epidemiol 2001;29(4):278–88.
9. Engelen L, de Wijk RA, Prinz JF, et al. The relation between saliva flow after different stimulations and the perception of flavor and texture attributes in custard desserts. Physiol Behav 2003;78(1):165–9.
10. Larsen MJ, Pearce EI. Saturation of human saliva with respect to calcium salts. Arch Oral Biol 2003;48(4):317–22.
11. Dodds MW, Johnson DA, Yeh CK. Health benefits of saliva: a review. J Dent 2005;33(3):223–33.
12. Dawes C, Kubieniec K. The effects of prolonged gum chewing on salivary flow rate and composition. Arch Oral Biol 2004;49(8):665–9.
13. Featherstone JD. Dental caries: a dynamic disease process. Aust Dent J 2008; 53(3):286–91.
14. Vitorino R, Calheiros-Lobo MJ, Duarte JA, et al. Salivary clinical data and dental caries susceptibility: is there a relationship? Bull Group Int Rech Sci Stomatol Odontol 2006;47(1):27–33.
15. Varma S, Banerjee A, Bartlett D. An in vivo investigation of associations between saliva properties, caries prevalence and potential lesion activity in an adult UK population. J Dent 2008;36(4):294–9.

16. Akpata ES, Al-Attar A, Sharma PN. Factors associated with severe caries among adults in Kuwait. Med Princ Pract 2009;18(2):93–9.
17. Ferguson DB. Salivary glands and saliva. In: Lavelle CLB, editor. Applied physiology of the mouth. Bristol (UK): John Wright; 1975. p. 145–79.
18. Peres RC, Camargo G, Mofatto LS, et al. Association of polymorphisms in the carbonic anhydrase 6 gene with salivary buffer capacity, dental plaque pH, and caries index in children aged 7–9 years. Pharmacogenomics J 2010;10(2):114–9.
19. Dawes C. An analysis of factors influencing diffusion from dental plaque into a moving film of saliva and the implications for caries. J Dent Res 1989; 68(11):1483–8.
20. Britse A, Lagerlöf F. The diluting effect of saliva on the sucrose concentration in different parts of the human mouth after a mouth-rinse with sucrose. Arch Oral Biol 1987;32(10):755–6.
21. Dawes C, Watanabe S, Biglow-Lecomte P, et al. Estimation of the velocity of the salivary film at some different locations in the mouth. J Dent Res 1989;68(11): 1479–82.
22. Suzuki A, Watanabe S, Ono Y, et al. Influence of the location of the parotid duct orifice on oral clearance. Arch Oral Biol 2009;54(3):274–8.
23. Brown LR, Dreizen S, Handler S, et al. Effect of radiation-induced xerostomia on human oral microflora. J Dent Res 1975;54(4):740–50.
24. Navazesh M. ADA Council on scientific Affairs and Division of Science. How can oral health care providers determine if patients have dry mouth? J Am Dent Assoc 2003;134(5):613–20.
25. Navazesh M, Mulligan RA, Kipnis V, et al. Comparison of whole saliva flow rates and mucin concentrations in healthy Caucasian young and aged adults. J Dent Res 1992;71(6):1275–8.
26. Percival RS, Challacombe SJ, Marsh PD. Flow rates of resting whole and stimulated parotid saliva in relation to age and gender. J Dent Res 1994;73(8):1416–20.
27. Heintze U, Birkhed D, Björn H. Secretion rate and buffer effect of resting and stimulated whole saliva as a function of age and sex. Swed Dent J 1983;7(6): 227–38.
28. Ben-Aryeh H, Shalev A, Szargel R, et al. The salivary flow rate and composition of whole and parotid resting and stimulated saliva in young and old healthy subjects. Biochem Med Metab Biol 1986;36(2):260–5.
29. Wynn RL, Meiller TF. Drugs and dry mouth. Gen Dent 2001;49(1):10–2 14.
30. Dreizen S, Brown LR, Daly TE, et al. Prevention of xerostomia-related dental caries in irradiated cancer patients. J Dent Res 1977;56(2):99–104.
31. Flink H, Tegelberg A, Lagerlöf F. Influence of the time of measurement of unstimulated human whole saliva on the diagnosis of hyposalivation. Arch Oral Biol 2005;50(6):553–9.
32. DePaola DP. Saliva: the precious body fluid. J Am Dent Assoc 2008;139(Suppl): 5S–6.
33. García-Godoy F, Hicks MJ. Maintaining the integrity of the enamel surface: the role of dental biofilm, saliva and preventive agents in enamel demineralization and remineralization. J Am Dent Assoc 2008;139(Suppl):25S–34.
34. Bolton RW, Hlava GL. Evaluation of salivary IgA antibodies to cariogenic microorganisms in children. Correlation with dental caries activity. J Dent Res 1982; 61(11):1225–8.
35. Gregory RL, Kindle JC, Hobbs LC, et al. Function of anti-*Streptococcus mutans* antibodies: inhibition of virulence factors and enzyme neutralization. Oral Microbiol Immunol 1990;5(4):181–8.

36. Rose PT, Gregory RL, Gfell LE, et al. IgA antibodies to *Streptococcus mutans* in caries-resistant and -susceptible children. Pediatr Dent 1994;16(4):272–5.
37. Sanui T, Gregory RL. Analysis of *Streptococcus mutans* biofilm proteins recognized by salivary immunoglobulin A. Oral Microbiol Immunol 2009; 24(5):361–8.
38. Moreno EC, Varughese K, Hay DI. Effect of human salivary proteins on the precipitation kinetics of calcium phosphate. Calcif Tissue Int 1979;28(1):7–16.
39. Hay DI, Pinsent BRW, Schram CJ, et al. The protective effect of calcium and phosphate ions against acid erosion of dental enamel and dentin. Br Dent J 1962;3:283–7.
40. Hay DI, Schluckebier SK, Moreno EC. Equilibrium dialysis and ultrafiltration studies of calcium and phosphate binding by human salivary proteins. Implications for salivary supersaturation with respect to calcium phosphate salts. Calcif Tissue Int 1982;34(6):531–8.
41. Aoba T, Moreno EC, Hay DI. Inhibition of apatite crystal growth by the amino-terminal segment of human salivary acidic proline-rich proteins. Calcif Tissue Int 1984;36(6):651–8.
42. Richardson CF, Johnsson M, Raj PA, et al. The influence of histatin-5 fragments on the mineralization of hydroxyapatite. Arch Oral Biol 1993;38(11):997–1002.
43. Johnsson M, Richardson CF, Bergey EJ, et al. The effects of human salivary cystatins and statherin on hydroxyapatite crystallization. Arch Oral Biol 1991;36(9): 631–6.
44. Mandel ID, Zorn M, Ruiz R, et al. The proteins and protein-bound carbohydrates of parotid saliva in caries-immune and caries-active adults. Arch Oral Biol 1965; 10(3):471–5.
45. Mandel ID, Bennick A. Quantitation of human salivary acidic proline-rich proteins in oral diseases. J Dent Res 1983;62(9):943–5.
46. Balekjian AY, Meyer TS, Montague ME, et al. Electrophoretic patterns of parotid fluid proteins from caries-resistant and caries-susceptible individuals. J Dent Res 1975;54(4):850–6.
47. Vitorino R, Lobo MJ, Duarte JR, et al. The role of salivary peptides in dental caries. Biomed Chromatogr 2005;19(3):214–22.
48. Rudney JD, Staikov RK, Johnson JD. Potential biomarkers of human salivary function: a modified proteomic approach. Arch Oral Biol 2009;54(1):91–100.
49. Van Nieuw Amerongen A, Bolscher JG, Veerman EC. Salivary proteins: protective and diagnostic value in cariology? Caries Res 2004;38(3):247–53.
50. Wong DT. Salivary diagnostics powered by nanotechnologies, proteomics and genomics. J Am Dent Assoc 2006;137(3):313–21.
51. Blicharz TM, Siqueira WL, Helmerhorst EJ, et al. Fiber-optic microsphere-based antibody array for the analysis of inflammatory cytokines in saliva. Anal Chem 2009;81(6):2106–14.
52. Scannapieco FA. Saliva-bacterium interactions in oral microbial ecology. Crit Rev Oral Biol Med 1994;5(3-4):203–48.
53. Skjørland KK, Rykke M, Sønju T. Rate of pellicle formation in vivo. Acta Odontol Scand 1995;53(6):358–62.
54. Vitkov L, Hannig M, Nekrashevych Y, et al. Supramolecular pellicle precursors. Eur J Oral Sci 2004;112(4):320–5.
55. Rolla G, Rykke M. Evidence for the presence of micelle-like protein globules in human saliva. Colloid Surface 1994;3:177–82.
56. Hannig M, Balz M. Protective properties of salivary pellicles from two different intraoral sites on enamel erosion. Caries Res 2001;35(2):142–8.

57. Hannig M. Ultrastructural investigation of pellicle morphogenesis at two different intraoral sites during a 24-h period. Clin Oral Investig 1999;3(2): 88–95.
58. Hannig M, Fiebiger M, Güntzer M, et al. Protective effect of the in situ formed short-term salivary pellicle. Arch Oral Biol 2004;49(11):903–10.
59. Hannig C, Hannig M, Attin T. Enzymes in the acquired enamel pellicle. Eur J Oral Sci 2005;113(1):2–13.
60. Lendenmann U, Grogan J, Oppenheim FG. Saliva and dental pellicle—a review. Adv Dent Res 2000;14:22–8.
61. Nieuw Amerongen AV, Oderkerk CH, Driessen AA. Role of mucins from human whole saliva in the protection of tooth enamel against demineralization in vitro. Caries Res 1987;21(4):297–309.
62. Featherstone JD, Behrman JM, Bell JE. Effect of whole saliva components on enamel demineralization in vitro. Crit Rev Oral Biol Med 1993;4(3-4): 357–62.
63. Kautsky MB, Featherstone JD. Effect of salivary components on dissolution rates of carbonated apatites. Caries Res 1993;27(5):373–7.
64. Duschner H, Hermann G, Walker R, et al. Erosion of dental enamel visualized by confocal laser scanning microscopy. In: Tooth wear and sensitivity. London: Martin Dunitz Ltd; 2000. p. 67–73.
65. Yao Y, Lamkin MS, Oppenheim FG. Pellicle precursor proteins: acidic proline-rich proteins, statherin, and histatins, and their crosslinking reaction by oral transglutaminase. J Dent Res 1999;78(11):1696–703.
66. Yao Y, Lamkin MS, Oppenheim FG. Pellicle precursor protein crosslinking characterization of an adduct between acidic proline-rich protein (PRP-1) and statherin generated by transglutaminase. J Dent Res 2000;79(4):930–8.
67. Zero DT. Etiology of dental erosion—extrinsic factors. Eur J Oral Sci 1996; 104(2):162–77.
68. Arends J, Schuthof J, Christoffersen J. Inhibition of enamel demineralization by albumin in vitro. Caries Res 1986;20(4):337–40.
69. Schüpbach P, Oppenheim FG, Lendenmann U, et al. Electron-microscopic demonstration of proline-rich proteins, statherin, and histatins in acquired enamel pellicles in vitro. Eur J Oral Sci 2001;109(1):60–8.
70. Bruvo M, Moe D, Kirkeby S, et al. Individual variations in protective effects of experimentally formed salivary pellicles. Caries Res 2009;43(3):163–70.
71. Siqueira WL, Zhang W, Helmerhorst EJ, et al. Identification of protein components in in vivo human acquired enamel pellicle using LC-ESI-MS/MS. J Proteome Res 2007;6(6):2152–60.
72. Siqueira WL, Oppenheim FG. Small molecular weight proteins/peptides present in the in vivo formed human acquired enamel pellicle. Arch Oral Biol 2009;54(5): 437–44.
73. Newbrun E. Dietary carbohydrates: their role in cariogenicity. Med Clin North Am 1979;63(5):1069–86.
74. Newbrun E. Sucrose in the dynamics of the carious process. Int Dent J 1982; 32(1):13–23.
75. van Houte J, Russo J. Variable colonization by oral streptococci in molar fissures of monoinfected gnotobiotic rats. Infect Immun 1986;52(2):620–2.
76. Gibbons RJ. Adherent interactions which may affect microbial ecology in the mouth. J Dent Res 1984;63(3):378–85.
77. Paes Leme AF, Koo H, Bellato CM, et al. The role of sucrose in cariogenic dental biofilm formation—new insight. J Dent Res 2006;85(10):878–87.

78. Zero DT, van Houte J, Russo J. The intra-oral effect on enamel demineralization of extracellular matrix material synthesized from sucrose by *Streptococcus mutans*. J Dent Res 1986;65(6):918–23.
79. Dibdin GH, Shellis RP. Physical and biochemical studies of *Streptococcus mutans* sediments suggest new factors linking the cariogenicity of plaque with its extracellular polysaccharide content. J Dent Res 1988;67(6):890–5.
80. Van Houte J, Russo J, Prostak KS. Increased pH-lowering ability of *Streptococcus mutans* cell masses associated with extracellular glucan-rich matrix material and the mechanisms involved. J Dent Res 1989;68(3):451–9.
81. Zero D, Fu J, Scott-Anne K, et al. Evaluation of fluoride dentifrices using a short-term intraoral remineralization model. J Dent Res 1994;73:272.
82. Zero DT. Sugars—the arch criminal? Caries Res 2004;38(3):277–85.
83. Bibby BG. Dental caries. Caries Res 1978;12(Suppl 1):3–6.
84. The National Health and Nutrition Examination Survey (NHANES). National Institute of Dental and Craniofacial Research Web site. Available at: http://www.nidcr.nih.gov/DataStatistics/FindDataByTopic/DentalCaries. Accessed March 23, 2010.
85. Burt BA. Relative consumption of sucrose and other sugars: has it been a factor in reduced caries experience? Caries Res 1993;27(Suppl 1):56–63.
86. Marshall TA. Chairside diet assessment of caries risk. J Am Dent Assoc 2009; 140(6):670–4.
87. Young RA. Biological apatite vs hydroxyapatite at the atomic level. Clin Orthop Relat Res 1975;113:249–62.
88. LeGeros RZ. Calcium phosphates in oral biology and medicine. Monogr Oral Sci 1991;15:1–201.
89. Ogaard B, Rölla G, Ruben J, et al. Microradiographic study of demineralization of shark enamel in a human caries model. Scand J Dent Res 1988;96(3):209–11.
90. LeGeros RZ, Tung MS. Chemical stability of carbonate- and fluoride-containing apatites. Caries Res 1983;17(5):419–29.
91. Losee FL, Bibby BG. Caries inhibition by trace elements other than fluorine. N Y State Dent J 1970;36(1):15–9.
92. Curzon ME, Crocker DC. Relationships of trace elements in human tooth enamel to dental caries. Arch Oral Biol 1978;23(8):647–53.
93. Featherstone JD. Diffusion phenomena and enamel caries development. In: Guggenheim B, editor. Cariology today. Zurich (Switzerland): Karger; 1983. p. 259–68.
94. Weatherell JA, Robinson C, Hallsworth AS. The concept of enamel resistance— a critical review. In: Guggenheim B, editor. Cariology today. Basel (Switzerland): Karger; 1984. p. 223–30.
95. Koulourides T. Implications of remineralization in the treatment of dental caries. Higashi Nippon Shigaku Zasshi 1986;5(1):1–20 87–97.
96. Carlos JP, Gittelsohn AM. Longitudinal studies of the natural history of caries. II. A life-table study of caries incidence in the permanent teeth. Arch Oral Biol 1965;10(5):739–51.
97. Kotsanos N, Darling AI. Influence of posteruptive age of enamel on its susceptibility to artificial caries. Caries Res 1991;25(4):241–50.
98. Bibby BG. Organic enamel material and caries. Caries Res 1971;5(4):305–22.
99. Zero DT. Dental caries process. Dent Clin North Am 1999;43:635–64.
100. Hoppenbrouwers PM, Driessens FC, Borggreven JM. The mineral solubility of human tooth roots. Arch Oral Biol 1987;32(5):319–22.
101. Wefel JS. Root caries histopathology and chemistry. Am J Dent 1994;7(5): 261–5.

102. Yoshiyama M, Sano H, Ebisu S, et al. Regional strengths of bonding agents to cervical sclerotic root dentin. J Dent Res 1996;75(6):1404–13.
103. Hara AT, Queiroz CS, Giannini M, et al. Influence of the mineral content and morphological pattern of artificial root caries lesion on composite resin bond strength. Eur J Oral Sci 2004;112(1):67–72.
104. Murchison DF, Charlton DG, Moore BK. Carbamide peroxide bleaching: effects on enamel surface hardness and bonding. Oper Dent 1992;17(5):181–5.
105. Flaitz CM, Hicks MJ. Effects of carbamide peroxide whitening agents on enamel surfaces and caries-like lesion formation: an SEM and polarized light microscopic in vitro study. ASDC J Dent Child 1996;63(4):249–56.
106. Rodrigues JA, Basting RT, Serra MC, et al. Effects of 10% carbamide peroxide bleaching materials on enamel microhardness. Am J Dent 2001;14(2):67–71.
107. Attin T, Kocabiyik M, Buchalla W, et al. Susceptibility of enamel surfaces to demineralization after application of fluoridated carbamide peroxide gels. Caries Res 2003;37(2):93–9.
108. Basting RT, Rodrigues AL Jr, Serra MC. The effects of seven carbamide peroxide bleaching agents on enamel microhardness over time. J Am Dent Assoc 2003;134(10):1335–42.
109. de Freitas PM, Turssi CP, Hara AT, et al. Monitoring of demineralized dentin microhardness throughout and after bleaching. Am J Dent 2004;17(5):342–6.
110. Arcari GM, Baratieri LN, Maia HP, et al. Influence of the duration of treatment using a 10% carbamide peroxide bleaching gel on dentin surface microhardness: an in situ study. Quintessence Int 2005;36(1):15–24.
111. Frysh H, Bowles WH, Baker F, et al. Effect of pH on hydrogen peroxide bleaching agents. J Esthet Dent 1995;7(3):130–3.
112. Pretty IA, Edgar WM, Higham SM. The effect of bleaching on enamel susceptibility to acid erosion and demineralisation. Br Dent J 2005;198(5):285–90.

The Chemistry of Caries: Remineralization and Demineralization Events with Direct Clinical Relevance

Carlos González-Cabezas, DDS, MSD, PhD

KEYWORDS

• Chemistry • Caries • Remineralization • Demineralization

This article discusses the main changes in tooth structure that occur during the formation, progression, and regression of caries lesions, with a particular focus on chemical and histologic events with direct relevance to the clinician.

Dental caries lesions arguably start to develop when demineralization of the tooth surface goes beyond the mineral exchanges that occur regularly between crystals at the surface of the tooth and the surrounding environment. Although, from the mechanistic point of view, these early events are important, from the clinical point of view early demineralization does not become relevant until it becomes clinically visible or detectable by other means (eg, radiography; **Fig. 1**). This clinical threshold is certain to change when new, more sensitive detection instruments become available. When conditions favorable for progression of the lesion continue for a significant time, these incipient noncavitated lesions continue to progress until the surface of the lesion collapses and a cavity is formed (**Fig. 2**). As the cavitated lesion continues to progress, the tooth can lose its vitality with a high risk of developing an infection beyond the tooth boundaries invading periapical tissues (**Fig. 3**).

THE DYNAMIC TOOTH SURFACE

Not all mineral loss from tooth structure is part of a pathologic process such as dental caries disease. Crystals at the tooth surface regularly go through natural periods of mineral loss (demineralization) and mineral gain (remineralization), particularly in surfaces covered by undisturbed (stagnant) biofilms (ie, dental plaque). Immediately

Department of Cariology, Restorative Sciences, and Endodontics, School of Dentistry, University of Michigan, 1011 North University B305, Ann Arbor, MI 48109-1078, USA
E-mail address: carlosgc@umich.edu

Dent Clin N Am 54 (2010) 469–478
doi:10.1016/j.cden.2010.03.004
0011-8532/10/$ – see front matter © 2010 Elsevier Inc. All rights reserved.

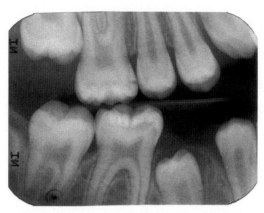

Fig. 1. Bitewing radiograph showing an approximal caries lesion in the mesial surface of a first maxillary molar.

after eruption into the oral cavity, teeth are colonized by oral bacteria that create conditions that, in combination with saliva, modify the composition of teeth surfaces, making them more resistant to dental caries. This process has been called posteruptive enamel maturation[1] and it is critically important for the caries process because it occurs in the tooth area with direct contact with the oral environment, where lesions start to develop.

Enamel surface crystal composition at eruption time has large amounts of carbonate, water, and magnesium, among other elements, and it is porous.[2,3] After undergoing many periods of demineralization and remineralization, the chemical composition and structure of surface enamel becomes more amorphous; less porous; contains less water, carbonates, and magnesium; and has increased amounts of fluoride and organic material.[4] These substitutions in the crystal surface are beneficial to the tooth surface because the new, matured tooth surface is less soluble and more resistant to caries challenges.[5,6]

A similar posteruptive maturation process is expected to occur on exposed root surfaces when the cementum or dentin is exposed to the oral environment after

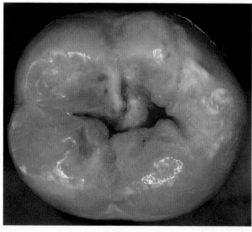

Fig. 2. A small cavitated caries lesion in the occlusal surface of a mandibular molar.

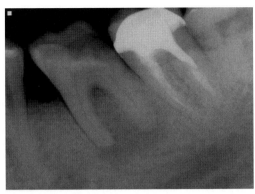

Fig. 3. Bitewing radiograph showing a periapical infection originated by an advanced caries lesion. (*Courtesy of* Dr Juan D. Saavedra.)

gingival recession. Cementum is typically lost quickly as a result of wear forces such as toothbrushing and scaling/root planning, and the highly porous and soluble newly exposed dentin undergoes similar demineralization and remineralization cycles, thus creating a much less porous dentinal surface containing larger amounts of minerals, particularly calcium, phosphate, and fluoride. This increase in crystal size and concentration significantly reduces the permeability and caries susceptibility of the root surface, as happens in enamel.

Crystals at the enamel and dentin/cementum surfaces covered by undisturbed biofilms are likely to continue having mineral exchanges for as long as the covering biofilms are able to create conditions of undersaturation and supersaturation with respect to the crystals. Undersaturation occurs mainly under acidic conditions by the loss of phosphate and hydroxyl ions that react with the hydrogen ions being produced by the metabolic activity of the covering biofilms in the presence of fermentable carbohydrates, particularly when they are frequently present; conditions commonly present in caries-active individuals.[7] In reaction to undersaturation conditions, minerals are released from multiple sources: saliva, bacteria, calculus, calcium-fluoride formations, and the tooth surface itself. After a period of time, saturation at the plaque fluid stabilizes and mineral loss stops. When enough minerals (mainly calcium, phosphate, and hydroxyl ions) are available in the solution surrounding the crystal increasing its saturation level, balance returns. At some point the pH can increase to a point at which supersaturation conditions can occur.[8] Under those conditions, the tendency of the solution is to precipitate minerals to return to saturated conditions. During this period of supersaturation, minerals can remineralize partially demineralized enamel crystals and, when supersaturation occurs for long periods of time, dental calculus can form, although protein inhibitors tend to prevent this from happening.[9] Therefore, although pH is the strongest determinant for saturation level leading to demineralization or remineralization under clinical conditions, it is not the only important factor because saturation is significantly affected by other factors such as the concentration of calcium and phosphate ions and the total ionic strength of plaque fluid.[8] This is clinically relevant because patients with significant decrease in salivary flow would have difficulty supplying enough minerals and buffering the fluid to maintain adequate saturation levels to maintain tooth surface integrity. There are other clinically relevant factors, such as the presence of calculus nearby, that also affect this process. Calculus crystals are less stable than those in tooth structure and therefore demineralize at higher saturation levels, releasing minerals into the plaque fluid protecting the tooth structure. Several clinical studies have shown an inverse relationship between caries and calculus.[10]

CARIES LESION FORMATION; ENAMEL

Under cariogenic conditions, the naturally increased tooth surface resistance is not enough to prevent the formation of a caries lesion. When, for a significant amount of time, the amount of minerals lost during those exchanges is larger than the amount of minerals gained, a caries lesion starts to develop in the enamel surface. The roughness and porosity of the tooth surface increases, presenting an eroded appearance at high magnification.[11] Increased porosity allows the development of a subsurface lesion, which is characteristic of caries lesions, distinguishing it from other types of demineralization such as dental erosion caused by stronger acids that promotes the loss of enamel structure layer by layer.

Caries lesions develop in the subsurface because of a series of unique phenomena that occur mainly around the lesion surface. Crystals at the tooth surface become more resistant to demineralization through the posteruptive maturation process and the formation of the lesion itself, leaving the subsurface crystals more susceptible to undersaturation conditions being created by the diffusion of hydrogen ions from plaque fluid. Moreover, the surface layer has better saturation conditions because, in addition to having access to ions coming from the body of the lesion and plaque fluid/saliva, it is also covered by the salivary pellicle, which acts as a diffusion barrier slowing down the outward diffusion of ions. These conditions increase saturation levels of calcium, phosphate, and fluoride at the surface, enhancing the probability of remineralization and reducing those of demineralization,[12] with the added consequence of the solution penetrating to the subsurface being much less saturated and with a reduced remineralization potential.[13] Consequently, fluoride has a much larger impact in the surface layer,[14] forming many crystal areas of less soluble fluoridated hydroxyapatite, which is more acid resistant and requires lower saturation levels before it starts to dissolve.[15] These conditions allow the caries lesion (demineralization secondary to acid penetration) to develop well into dentin without breakage of the surface, and it is probably bacteria free in most cases because bacteria are physically too large to fit into the diffusion spaces of a seemingly intact surface layer.

Mineral surfaces are covered with organic material that restricts ion exchange, limiting the rate of demineralization and remineralization by acting as a diffusion barrier for mineral exchanges. Some laboratory evidence suggests that the net result of this restriction is enhanced protection by a reduction in the amount of hydrogen ions going in and the amount of calcium and phosphate going out, increasing the saturation level at those specific locations.[16] Furthermore, fluoride ions are likely to concentrate at those locations and only sub–parts per million (ppm) levels of fluoride near the crystal are needed to significantly affect saturation levels.[13,17] Therefore, lesion progression is not only determined by the level of undersaturation but also by the ability of the ions to diffuse in and out of the lesion, which has been shown to be slow.[18]

Large portions of the noncavitated lesion can be remineralized if the saturation condition cycle shifts to conditions in which more mineral is gained than lost. Under these favorable conditions, remineralization of the lesion surface is more likely to occur first, leading to the blockage of the communication channels that allowed the demineralization of the subsurface of the lesion. These particular dynamics lead to the formation of a remineralized surface that is highly resistance to demineralization (probably more resistant than sound enamel[19]), leaving a sealed, partially demineralized subsurface lesion.[20] Although this situation might concern some clinicians, many noncavitated caries lesions develop and become arrested naturally, with no detrimental clinical consequences. As long the saturation conditions in the biofilms covering those lesions do not return to cariogenicity, those lesions do not progress and teeth are fully functional. Many early noncavitated (white and brown spot) lesions will continue to be visible clinically and radiographically after remineralization because most of the detection signal comes from the body of the lesion, where changes in its light scattering and radiolucency are unlikely because of its limited remineralization potential (**Fig. 4**).

Caries lesions develop following the shape of the undisturbed biofilms covering the tooth surface where the lesion is developing. For example, early caries lesions in the proximal surfaces typically are curved following the cervical margin of the contact. In occlusal surfaces, where most of the caries lesions develop, most lesions develop at the entrance of fissures and fossae and the bottom of wider ones. These are areas of higher risk because of their limited salivary access and propensity to accumulate undisturbed biofilms. Therefore, conditions leading to the growth of undisturbed biofilms create site-specific high-risk situations that might lead to the development of caries lesions. Good examples are occlusal surfaces of erupting teeth that are not yet fully functional in mastication and are easily covered by significant amounts of undisturbed biofilm, greatly increasing the risk for lesion development[21,22] or large gaps between dental restorations and tooth structure in approximal surfaces, also promoting the accumulation of undisturbed biofilm and consequently increasing the risk of developing secondary caries lesions.[23]

CARIES LESION FORMATION; DENTIN

During the development of incipient (noncavitated) lesions, dentin undergoes significant changes in reaction to acids diffusing through the demineralized enamel from the overlaying biofilms. These changes occur at early stages as a result of the high diffusibility of the enamel to small-chain organic acids. The demineralization/remineralization thermodynamics in dentin are similar to those in enamel, but with some unique characteristics. Dentinal crystals are smaller and more reactive than those in enamel. The dental pulp reacts to intraoral events even when the enamel is intact; for example, in cases of trauma or excessive occlusal forces. The caries process also stimulates a reaction that is expressed in the mineralization of the intratubular space, known as dentinal sclerosis. During the initial phases of lesion formation, minerals from the less mineralized interdentinal dentin demineralize and precipitatation of some of these

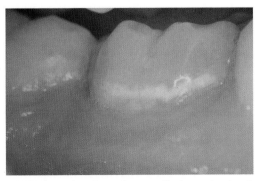

Fig. 4. A caries lesion in the buccal surface of a mandibular molar that has been arrested for more than 30 years.

minerals occurs in the dentinal tubule lumens in the form of hydroxyapatite and whit-lockite crystals, reducing permeability of the dentin.[24] These events are modulated by the continuous fluid pressure gradient toward the outside coming from the dental pulp.[25] The tubular sclerosis that starts to develop before clear enamel demineraliza-tion has reached the dentinoenamel junction (DEJ) is the first sign of dentinal reaction to the caries process that can be detected at low microscopic magnification; other biochemical and molecular reactions leading to the sclerosis start happening at earlier stages. As the lesion continues to progress, this process continues and the more mineralized peritubular dentin starts to demineralize, widening the opening of the dentinal tubules and increasing the diffusion rate. The dental pulp also reacts by increasing the deposition of dentin around the pulp (tertiary or reactive dentin), poten-tially protecting it from damage.[26,27] These events occur without significant direct bacterial invasion; they are triggered by bacterial products.[28]

It is commonly believed that caries lesions spread laterally after reaching the DEJ, but the available evidence suggests that lesions follow the axial direction of the enamel lesion,[29] although lateral spread might happen after cavitation.[30] Because of its diffu-sion-related dynamics, lesions follow the path of easier diffusion, which typically is the direction of the enamel rods and the dentinal tubules. Lesions can advance to signif-icant levels of demineralization in the dentin without cavitation of the surface.[31] Because the lesion progresses following the enamel rods, occlusal lesions are typi-cally narrower at the enamel surface than at the DEJ, creating a lesion having an inverted-cone shape.[29] In cases in which an initial small cavitation is developed at those locations, conditions are created for the rapid development of a hidden lesion.

CARIES LESION FORMATION: CAVITATION

At some point, the three-dimensional structure of a lesion is not able to withstand the stresses created by external forces coming from mastication, brushing, or even a dental explorer used improperly, and the surface collapses, creating an irreversible cavitation. Most cavitations, particularly at the early stages, create a protective envi-ronment for the dental biofilms in which bacteria grow undisturbed, creating a cario-genic environment. Diffusion of acids from the biofilm continues through the previously expanded diffusion pathways, and biofilm thickness reduces the potential remineral-izing effect of saliva minerals and fluoride. Bacteria soon start invading enamel and dentin, accelerating the progression of the lesion. With the opening of pathways, bacteria are able to invade deep into the dentinal lumens, increasing the speed of progression and the likelihood of injuring the pulp. After significant bacterial invasion, organic destruction can be observed due to the proteolytic action of bacterial enzymes mainly on the collagen matrix, resulting in an increase of the cavity size and further biofilm invasion.

The dentinal lesion presents different levels of demineralization, having the most advanced areas closer to the biofilm growing on the surface of the cavity. Areas next to the invading biofilm are highly demineralized, with organic material in advanced levels of destruction and with high levels of bacteria present. The destruc-tion level diminishes toward the areas in the forefront of the lesion. These 2 grossly defined zones of carious dentin have previously been defined as affected and infected dentin with the intention of providing some clinical guidelines for carious tissue removal.[32] These different zones have characteristically different hardness levels that would be detected clinically by the careful clinician,[33] and these levels have been related to the level of caries activity.[34] Removal of highly infected dentin and leaving the affected layer is a reasonable clinical goal because the affected dentin is remineralizable because the collagen still retains its cross-linkage with enough nucleating minerals to permit remineralization.[35] Excessive removal of affected dentin commonly occurs when dentists try to reach for the hardness of sound dentin. Furthermore, some clinical data suggest that even removal of infected dentin might not be necessary if the lesion can be sealed[36] and has potential for remineralization.[37,38]

REMINERALIZATION

Remineralization of active noncavitated lesions should be an expected outcome of any caries management therapy. Remineralization of noncavitated lesions has been reported since the beginning of the twentieth century, when demineralized enamel was observed to harden in the presence of saliva.[39] Several decades later, clinical studies demonstrated that noncavitated caries lesions can be repaired by saliva, in particular when plaque covering the lesion is removed regularly in combination with fluoride treatments.[40–42] Partially demineralized enamel and dentin apatite crystals can be remineralized to almost their original size under optimal laboratory conditions. However, under clinical conditions most of the remineralization occurs at the surface, leaving a sealed subsurface underneath[18] for reasons discussed earlier. This remineralized enamel surface is different from the original in its composition and structure, and it is more resistant to demineralization than sound enamel.[19]

Remineralization needs bioavailable calcium and phosphate, and it is greatly enhanced by the presence of fluoride even at sub-ppm levels. Laboratory data suggest that the levels of fluoride needed for established noncavitated lesions might be greater than those to prevent lesion formation.[13] However, remineralization is not possible after the mineral phase if its nucleation sites are lost completely. Furthermore, because creating conditions of saturation or supersaturation requires the supply of significant amounts of minerals from saliva, patients with reduced salivary flow are difficult to manage and require extreme preventive measures in some cases, when salivary flow recovery is not an option.

Many clinicians quickly associate any dentinal involvement with operative treatment management needs. However, as described earlier, dentinal involvement is complex, and management of the lesion involves many options. Even cavitated lesions can arrest if cariogenic conditions change.[43] Although most cavitated lesions protect biofilms from disturbing forces enhancing the cariogenic conditions and require operative therapy to control the disease, this is not always the case. For example, in advanced lesions with most cavity walls lost the exposed tooth, mainly dentin, is self-cleansable and biofilms do not accumulate easily on the dentin surface for long periods of time, creating conditions leading to lesion remineralization and arrestment. A good example of the potential of dentinal lesion arrestment can be observed in root surface caries lesions that can be remineralized by brushing with fluoridated toothpastes.[44,45] Advanced arrested lesions might need restorative treatment to restore function or esthetics.

Understanding that noncavitated caries lesions can be arrested and reversed has led to a paradigm change for caries management. Consequently, significant amount of caries research has been focused on developing new and better remineralizing therapies. Fluoride continues to be considered the most important therapy available today to promote lesion remineralization. Different calcium-based formulations are being developed and commercialized, and early data suggest that they might have remineralizing properties, but these products are still in developmental phases with insufficient clinical evidence,[46] and so far none of them have been shown to be more effective than fluoride. It is likely that the development of new therapies in combination with the enhancement of current management protocols will transform the standard of care for caries prevention and management.

SUMMARY

Dental caries is a site-specific disease that undergoes many cycles of demineralization and remineralization during lesion development. Because of its developmental characteristics dynamics, the caries lesion can be arrested and even repaired at its early stages without operative intervention by increasing the net mineral gain during the demineralization and remineralization cycles. This result can be accomplished by reducing the effect of etiological factors such as cariogenic biofilms and diet, and increasing the efficacy of remineralizing agents such as saliva and fluoride.

REFERENCES

1. Francis MD, Briner WW. The development and regression of hypomineralized areas of rat molars. Arch Oral Biol 1966;11(3):349–54.
2. Crabb HS. The porous outer enamel of unerupted human premolars. Caries Res 1976;10(1):1–7.
3. Driessens FC, Heijligers HJ, Borggreven JM, et al. Posteruptive maturation of tooth enamel studied with the electron microprobe. Caries Res 1985;19(5):390–5.
4. Brudevold F, Steadman LT, Smith FA. Inorganic and organic components of tooth structure. Ann N Y Acad Sci 1960;85:110–32.
5. Kidd EA, Richards A, Thylstrup A, et al. The susceptibility of 'young' and 'old' human enamel to artificial caries in vitro. Caries Res 1984;18(3):226–30.
6. Kotsanos N, Darling AI. Influence of posteruptive age of enamel on its susceptibility to artificial caries. Caries Res 1991;25(4):241–50.
7. Margolis HC, Zhang YP, van Houte J, et al. Effect of sucrose concentration on the cariogenic potential of pooled plaque fluid from caries-free and caries-positive individuals. Caries Res 1993;27(6):467–73.
8. Margolis HC, Moreno EC. Composition and cariogenic potential of dental plaque fluid. Crit Rev Oral Biol Med 1994;5(1):1–25.
9. Moreno EC, Varughese K, Hay DI. Effect of human salivary proteins on the precipitation kinetics of calcium phosphate. Calcif Tissue Int 1979;28(1):7–16.
10. Duckworth RM. On the relationship between calculus and caries. In: Duckworth RM, editor, The teeth and their environment, vol. 19. Basel (Switzerland): Karger; 2006. p. 1–28.
11. Holmen L, Thylstrup A, Ogaard B, et al. A scanning electron microscopic study of progressive stages of enamel caries in vivo. Caries Res 1985;19(4):355–67.
12. Weatherell JA, Robinson C, Hallsworth AS. The concept of enamel resistance - a critical review. In: Guggenheim B, editor. Cariology today. Basel (Switzerland): Karger; 1984. p. 223–30.
13. Yamazaki H, Litman A, Margolis HC. Effect of fluoride on artificial caries lesion progression and repair in human enamel: regulation of mineral deposition and dissolution under in vivo-like conditions. Arch Oral Biol 2007;52(2):110–20.
14. Pearce EI, Coote GE, Larsen MJ. The distribution of fluoride in carious human enamel. J Dent Res 1995;74(11):1775–82.
15. Margolis HC, Moreno EC, Murphy BJ. Effect of low levels of fluoride in solution on enamel demineralization in vitro. J Dent Res 1986;65(1):23–9.
16. Aoba T, Moreno EC, Hay DI. Inhibition of apatite crystal growth by the amino-terminal segment of human salivary acidic proline-rich proteins. Calcif Tissue Int 1984;36(6):651–8.

17. ten Cate JM, Duijsters PP. Influence of fluoride in solution on tooth demineralization. I. Chemical data. Caries Res 1983;17(3):193–9.
18. Larsen MJ, Fejerskov O. Chemical and structural challenges in remineralization of dental enamel lesions. Scand J Dent Res 1989;97(4):285–96.
19. Iijima Y, Takagi O. In situ acid resistance of in vivo formed white spot lesions. Caries Res 2000;34(5):388–94.
20. Iijima Y, Takagi O, Ruben J, et al. In vitro remineralization of in vivo and in vitro formed enamel lesions. Caries Res 1999;33(3):206–13.
21. Carvalho JC, Ekstrand KR, Thylstrup A. Dental plaque and caries on occlusal surfaces of first permanent molars in relation to stage of eruption. J Dent Res 1989;68(5):773–9.
22. Carvalho JC, Thylstrup A, Ekstrand KR. Results after 3 years of non-operative occlusal caries treatment of erupting permanent first molars. Community Dent Oral Epidemiol 1992;20(4):187–92.
23. Totiam P, Gonzalez-Cabezas C, Fontana MR, et al. A new in vitro model to study the relationship of gap size and secondary caries. Caries Res 2007;41(6):467–73.
24. Stanley HR, Pereira JC, Spiegel E, et al. The detection and prevalence of reactive and physiologic sclerotic dentin, reparative dentin and dead tracts beneath various types of dental lesions according to tooth surface and age. J Oral Pathol 1983;12(4):257–89.
25. Shellis RP. Effects of a supersaturated pulpal fluid on the formation of caries-like lesions on the roots of human teeth. Caries Res 1994;28(1):14–20.
26. Frank RM, Voegel JC. Ultrastructure of the human odontoblast process and its mineralisation during dental caries. Caries Res 1980;14(6):367–80.
27. Bjorndal L. Presence or absence of tertiary dentinogenesis in relation to caries progression. Adv Dent Res 2001;15:80–3.
28. Ratledge DK, Kidd EA, Beighton D. A clinical and microbiological study of approximal carious lesions. Part 2: efficacy of caries removal following tunnel and class II cavity preparations. Caries Res 2001;35(1):8–11.
29. Bjorndal L, Mjor IA. Pulp-dentin biology in restorative dentistry. Part 4: dental caries–characteristics of lesions and pulpal reactions. Quintessence Int 2001; 32(9):717–36.
30. Ekstrand KR, Ricketts DN, Kidd EA. Do occlusal carious lesions spread laterally at the enamel-dentin junction? A histolopathological study. Clin Oral Investig 1998;2(1):15–20.
31. Pitts NB, Rimmer PA. An in vivo comparison of radiographic and directly assessed clinical caries status of posterior approximal surfaces in primary and permanent teeth. Caries Res 1992;26(2):146–52.
32. Fusayama T, Terachima S. Differentiation of two layers of carious dentin by staining. J Dent Res 1972;51(3):866.
33. Ogawa K, Yamashita Y, Ichijo T, et al. The ultrastructure and hardness of the transparent layer of human carious dentin. J Dent Res 1983;62(1):7–10.
34. Zheng L, Hilton JF, Habelitz S, et al. Dentin caries activity status related to hardness and elasticity. Eur J Oral Sci 2003;111(3):243–52.
35. Kuboki Y, Ohgushi K, Fusayama T. Collagen biochemistry of the two layers of carious dentin. J Dent Res 1977;56(10):1233–7.
36. Mertz-Fairhurst EJ, Curtis JW Jr, Ergle JW, et al. Ultraconservative and cariostatic sealed restorations: results at year 10. J Am Dent Assoc 1998;129(1):55–66.
37. Maltz M, de Oliveira EF, Fontanella V, et al. A clinical, microbiologic, and radiographic study of deep caries lesions after incomplete caries removal. Quintessence Int 2002;33(2):151–9.

38. ten Cate JM. Remineralization of caries lesions extending into dentin. J Dent Res 2001;80(5):1407–11.
39. Head JA. A study on saliva and its action on tooth enamel in reference to its hardening and softening. JAMA 1912;59:2118–22.
40. von der Fehr FR. Maturation and remineralisation of enamel. Adv Fluorine Res 1965;3:83–95.
41. Backer Dirks O. Posteruptive changes in dental enamel. J Dent Res 1966; 45(Suppl 3):503–11.
42. Loe H, Von der Fehr FR, Schiott CR. Inhibition of experimental caries by plaque prevention. The effect of chlorhexidine mouthrinses. Scand J Dent Res 1972; 80(1):1–9.
43. Levine RS. The microradiographic features of dentine caries. Observations on 200 lesions. Br Dent J 1974;137(8):301–6.
44. Nyvad B, ten Cate JM, Fejerskov O. Arrest of root surface caries in situ. J Dent Res 1997;76(12):1845–53.
45. Baysan A, Lynch E, Ellwood R, et al. Reversal of primary root caries using dentifrices containing 5,000 and 1,100 ppm fluoride. Caries Res 2001;35(1):41–6.
46. Azarpazhooh A, Limeback H. Clinical efficacy of casein derivatives: a systematic review of the literature. J Am Dent Assoc 2008;139(7):915–24 [quiz: 994–5].

Detection Activity Assessment and Diagnosis of Dental Caries Lesions

Mariana M. Braga, DDS, PhD[a], Fausto M. Mendes, DDS, MS, PhD[a],
Kim R. Ekstrand, DDS, PhD[b],*

KEYWORDS

- Dental caries • Caries indices • Caries detection
- ICDAS • Radiographic methods • Caries activity

The word diagnosis (plural, diagnoses) is derived from the Greek "dia" meaning "through" and "gnosis" meaning "knowledge".[1] Thus, "to diagnose" implies that it is only through knowledge about the disease that a diagnosis can be established. Diagnosis can be a complicated process.[1,2]

Caries disease diagnosis is not the classical hypothetical-deductive process that diagnosis often is in the medical world.[3] When a patient visits a doctor, the patient tells his or her symptoms to the doctor. The doctor examines the patient and based on his diagnostic hypotheses (knowledge), the doctor chooses the diagnosis that best fits the patient's signs and symptoms and the treatment that offers the best prognosis for the patient. This systematic approach permits thinking about all the possibilities available to solve the patient's problem. Dentists, on the other hand, usually examine their patients thinking about how they will treat the patients' teeth, rather than thinking about the condition (diagnoses) of the patients' teeth. Thus, a great deal of information relevant to disease diagnosis can be lost and some treatment options (usually more conservative alternatives) can be underestimated during the final clinical decision making.[3]

The examination and evaluation of carious lesions has traditionally been limited to physical criteria such as size, depth, and presence or absence of cavitation. The term for this is caries lesion detection.[2,4–6] Caries lesion activity assessment is different from caries lesion detection. The assessment of lesion activity is, together with lesion detection, essential to arrive at the disease diagnosis and the appropriate

[a] Department of Pediatric Dentistry, Faculdade de Odontologia da Universidade de São Paulo, Avenida Professor Lineu Prestes 2227, São Paulo, SP 05508-900, Brazil
[b] Department of Cariology and Endodontics, School of Dentistry, Faculty of Health Sciences, University of Copenhagen, 20 Nörre alle, DK-2200, Copenhagen N, Denmark
* Corresponding author.
E-mail address: kim@odont.ku.dk

Dent Clin N Am 54 (2010) 479–493
doi:10.1016/j.cden.2010.03.006
0011-8532/10/$ – see front matter © 2010 Elsevier Inc. All rights reserved.

clinical treatment decision.[2,4–6] In addition to caries lesion detection, lesion or disease activity assessment must also consider etiologic factor evaluations, such as oral hygiene, count of cariogenic micro-organisms in plaque and saliva, use of fluoride, sugar intake, and also some socioeconomic aspects, such as family income and parents' level of education.[2,6,7] It becomes evident that caries disease diagnosis is a difficult task. This article focuses on caries lesion detection including evaluation of caries lesion severity. The authors explore conventional and advanced/modern methods of caries lesion detection, their properties, limitations, and indications. They discuss the interpretation of the results obtained by these methods. Finally, parameters to be used for assessing lesion activity in order to reach a final caries disease diagnosis and relate the treatment decision to this diagnosis are discussed. As caries risk assessment is covered in another article (see the article by Young and Featherstone elsewhere in this issue), the focus of attention in this article is on caries lesions (signs) and the related treatment decisions.

VISUAL INSPECTION

Visual examination is the most commonly used method for detecting caries lesions, because it is an easy technique that is routinely performed in clinical practice.[8] Visual examination has presented high specificity (proportion of sound sites correctly identified), but low sensitivity (proportion of carious sites correctly identified), and low reproducibility[9]; the latter because of its subjective nature.

The use of detailed visual indices, however, may improve sensitivity and be an important factor in minimizing the examiner's interpretation of the clinical characteristics of a lesion, and thus improve reproducibility. Such indices may also describe the characteristics of all clinically relevant stages in the caries disease process, making them a cost-effective method of recording caries lesions. The use of indices has permitted early caries signs to be detected and recorded in a reliable and accurate way in visual examination.[10–16] However, initial caries lesion stages have generated most of the disagreements between examiners in several studies, and their evaluation demands more training and more time for examination.[17]

A review found 29 different visual criteria for detecting caries lesions.[18] Each system has its own particularities and methodology of teeth/surface evaluation.[11,18] Only about half of the technologies recommend teeth to be cleaned and/or dried before the examination process (14 criteria), which if not included will increase the risk of missing lesions (**Fig. 1**). Further, caries lesion activity assessment is not considered by most of these indices, which is a limitation in clinical practice. In addition, some indices recommend tactile examination to be performed in conjunction with visual examination, and this has been considered questionable. Probing-related surface defects, enlargements, and damage to dental surfaces have been observed on surfaces with initial carious lesions (see **Fig. 1**D and E).[19,20] Some previous reviews have shown inconclusive results with regard to tactile examination performance, and a lack of information concerning the examiner's training and manner of using the explorer (to remove plaque, to gently probe).[9,18] The most recent trend is the use of the probe to evaluate enamel surface texture (smooth or rough for enamel lesions; hard or soft dentine for dentinal lesions). Another recommendation is evaluation of the presence of discontinuities in enamel or microcavitations by using the WHO probe, which is ball-ended with a sphere presenting 0.5 mm in the extremity, allowing this kind of evaluation.

In an attempt to propose an internationally accepted caries detection system, a new index for caries diagnosis, the International and Caries Detection Assessment System, was created in 2002 by a group of cariologists and epidemiologists, based on visual

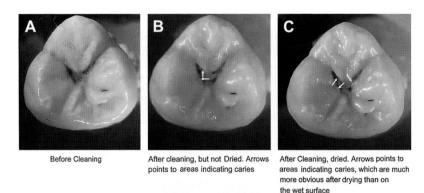

Before Cleaning | After cleaning, but not Dried. Arrows points to areas indicating caries | After Cleaning, dried. Arrows points to areas indicating caries, which are much more obvious after drying than on the wet surface

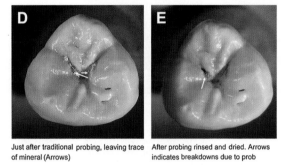

Just after traditional probing, leaving trace of mineral (Arrows) | After probing rinsed and dried. Arrows indicates breakdowns due to prob

Fig. 1. (*A–E*) Examples showing the benefit of cleaning and drying to detect caries (*A–C*) and the harmful effect of probing with a sharp explorer (*D, E*).

examination aided by a WHO probe. The short name of this system is ICDAS.[21] This system is a modification of a previous visually ranked caries lesion scoring system that has been shown to detect occlusal lesions in permanent teeth and to assess their depth with acceptable accuracy and reproducibility.[13,22]

ICDAS is a 2-digit identification system (X-Y). Firstly, the status of the surfaces is recorded as unrestored, sealed, restored, or crowned. After that, a second code is attributed (Y). This code ranges from measurement of first visual changes in the enamel to extensive cavitation. The description and examples of each code are presented in **Fig. 2**.[23] Before examination, teeth have to be carefully cleaned and examinations must be performed with light illumination, an air syringe, plane buccal mirror and, if necessary, a WHO periodontal probe.

The validity of ICDAS has been tested and expressed in many ways. For example, ICDAS has presented content validity (the system is comprehensible for describing and measuring different degrees of severity of caries lesions). Further, a significant correlation with lesion depth in the histologic examination has been shown.[15,22,24,25] Criterion validity of ICDAS, which means how well the system is correlated with the actual severity of the caries lesions, was also observed in vitro for permanent and primary teeth. Its performance has varied from moderate to good. In terms of figures, the sensitivity for occlusal surfaces have varied from 0.63 to 0.82 and specificity from 0.63 to 0.94.[15,22,24–27]

In primary teeth, ICDAS cannot distinguish accurately between lesions related to the outer or inner half of the enamel[15]; this can be done fairly accurately in permanent teeth. One explanation for this difference in performance is that the enamel in primary teeth is much thinner compared with permanent enamel.[28,29]

Score	Criteria
0	No or slight change in enamel translucency after prolonged air drying (5s)
1	First visual change in enamel (seen only after prolonged air drying or restricted to within the confines of a pit or fissure
2	Distinct visual changes in enamel
3	Localized enamel breakdown in opaque or discoloured enamel (without visual signs of dentinal involvement)
4	Underlying dark shadow from dentine
5	Distinct cavity with visible dentin
6	Extensive distinct cavity with visible dentin (involving more than half of the surface)

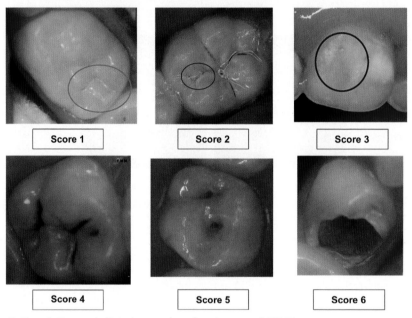

Score 1   Score 2   Score 3

Score 4   Score 5   Score 6

Fig. 2. Description and clinical examples of each score of ICDAS.

Few studies have been performed in proximal surfaces using ICDAS. In general, the interexaminer reproducibility has been similar to that observed for occlusal surfaces.[10,16,27] The system has presented good performance (high sensitivity and specificity) for in vitro conditions.[10,27] However, its sensitivity has been low for proximal caries in vivo, whereas the specificity has been high, even when considering the noncavitated threshold.[16] These properties should encourage the use of ICDAS also in proximal caries detection, although other additional methods should be added to improve sensitivity on these surfaces.

Initially, ICDAS was devised as a detection system for primary caries. Adjunct criteria have recently been devised for activity assessment. Thus, the system can be used for caries lesion activity assessment (LAA) also. The LAA is based on the combined knowledge of clinical appearance (ICDAS) of the lesion, whether or not the lesion is in a plaque stagnation area, and the tactile sensation when a ball-ended WHO probe is gently drawn across the surface of the tooth. Such criteria related to activity receive an individual score (points) based on predictive value in determining activity status, and the sum of these points is judged based on a cut-off point

(**Table 1**).[24] These individual criteria have presented moderate to good intra- and inter-examiner reproducibility values,[15,24] as well as good reproducibility results for the system overall.[15] This system also presented construct validity (ie, the system is able to reflect theoretical concepts regarding the caries process).[24]

Two studies have already used the ICDAS+LAA system in caries activity assessment.[30,31] One of these studies concluded that areas of plaque stagnation were more associated with caries lesion activity status than surface texture.[30] The other study used the system successfully to verify an association between caries lesion activity and some biologic parameters.[31] Results have suggested that the use of this system could overestimate caries lesion activity status for primary teeth, because cavitated lesions invariably would be considered active, which is not certain in all cases. However, validity parameters could be improved if new cut-off points were adopted. New studies should be encouraged to reevaluate the importance attributed to each clinical parameter or to revise the cut-off point used to classify caries lesion activity in primary teeth.

Using the ICDAS in combination with the LAA criteria described here, it is possible to detect a lesion, estimate its depth or severity, and assess its activity, which are all fundamental prerequisites for the diagnosis and management of the individual lesion.[24,32]

Nyvad's System

Nyvad's system (**Table 2**) is another reliable option for activity assessment of noncavitated and cavitated caries lesions.[14,15] This system has presented construct and predictive validity (the different status of caries lesions can be predictive of different outcomes) concerning caries lesion activity status.[14] According to this system, a score can be attributed to all observed characteristics of the lesion, eventually classifying the lesion as inactive or active. If a lesion presents at least 1 feature compatible to an active lesion, the examiner should classify the lesion as active. The original system used plaque as an indicator for caries lesion activity and used standard probes to assess roughness. Some recent studies have performed examinations using Nyvad's scoring

Table 1
Description of the method for lesion activity assessment proposed to be used after evaluation with ICDAS

Criterion	Description	Activity Score
Clinical parameter 1 (Visual appearance: severity score)		
ICDAS score 1, 2 (brown lesions)		1
ICDAS score 1, 2 (white lesions)		3
ICDAS score 3, 4, 5, or 6		4
Clinical parameter 2 (Plaque stagnation)		
Plaque stagnation area (PSA)	Plaque stagnation area (PSA) along the gingival, below or above the contact area on proximal surfaces, entrance to the pits and fissures and cavities with irregular borders	3
Non plaque stagnation area (non-PSA)	Flat pits and fissures	1
Clinical parameter 3 (Surface texture)		
Rough or soft surface on gentle probing		4
Smooth or hard surface on gentle probing		2

From Ekstrand KR, Martignon S, Ricketts DJ, et al. Detection and activity assessment of primary coronal caries lesions: a methodologic study. Oper Dent 2007;32(3):225–35; with permission.

Table 2
Description of the scores in the Nyvad system

Score	Category	Criteria
0	Sound	Normal enamel translucency and texture (slight staining allowed in otherwise sound fissure)
1	Active caries (intact surface)	Surface of enamel is whitish/yellowish, opaque with loss of luster; feels rough when the tip of the probe is moved gently across the surface; generally covered with plaque. No clinically detectable loss of substance. Intact fissure morphology; lesion extending along the walls of the fissure
2	Active caries (surface discontinuity)	Same criteria as score 1. Localized surface defect (microcavity) in enamel only. No undermined enamel or softened floor detectable with the explorer
	Active caries (cavity)	Enamel/dentine cavity easily visible with the naked eye; surface of the cavity feels soft or leathery on gentle probing. There may or may not be pulpal involvement
4	Inactive caries (intact surface)	Surface of enamel is whitish, brownish, or black. Enamel may be shiny and feel hard and smooth when the tip of the probe is moved gently across the surface. No clinically detectable loss of substance. Intact fissure morphology; lesion extending along the walls of the fissure
5	Inactive caries (surface discontinuity)	Same criteria as score 4. Localized surface defect (microcavity) in enamel only. No undermined enamel or softened floor detectable with the explorer
6	Inactive caries (cavity)	Enamel/dentine cavity easily visible with the naked eye; surface of the cavity feels shiny and feels hard on gentle probing. No pulpal involvement
7	Filling (sound surface)	
8	Filling + active caries	Caries lesion may be cavitated or noncavitated
9	Filling + inactive caries	Caries lesion may be cavitated or noncavitated

criteria exactly as published. However, to standardize the methodology used in the examinations, the Nyvad system was modified in several ways compared with the original version, adopting inspection after prophylaxis and the use of the WHO probe.[15]

Although it was not its original purpose, the Nyvad index worked well in assessing the depth of lesions on primary teeth.[15] As observed for ICDAS, microcavities, that is, cavitation limited to enamel (scores 2 and 5 in the Nyvad system, score 3 in ICDAS), usually involve dentin demineralization in primary teeth.[15]

It is inherent that visual examination must be the main method for caries detection, whereas the methods described below tend to act as adjuncts, depending on the purpose of the examination. It is worth emphasizing that visual examination is the only effective method available to assess caries lesion activity.[2,14,32,33] The use of the indices to assess caries lesion activity described in this article ,should be considered in daily clinical practice.

ADDITIONAL METHODS TO DETECT CARIES LESIONS
Radiographic Methods

In permanent teeth, sensitivity values of visual examination obtained in clinical studies in detecting proximal caries lesions have been around 0.30.[34,35] A study by Novaes and colleagues[16] obtained similar figures in detecting cavitated lesions in the proximal surfaces of primary molars. Therefore, around 70% of cavitated caries lesions would be missed using visual inspection.

The use of a bitewing radiography as an adjunct to the clinical examination could permit more sensitive detection of proximal and occlusal caries lesions in dentin and a better estimation of the lesion depth than the visual inspection performed alone. Moreover, the monitoring of caries lesions could be more reliable and accurate than using the conventional clinical examination alone.[36]

Bitewing projection is the most appropriate radiographic technique for caries detection. This technique requires a film-holder with a wing for the patient to bite. A good technique is necessary to avoid overlapping surfaces, cone cuts, and missing surfaces. In such conditions, the bitewing radiographs provide valuable information to complete the clinical diagnosis.[36]

Some disadvantages, however, are present and must be considered when making treatment decisions, mainly on proximal surfaces. First, radiographic images underestimate the actual lesion depth (measured histologically), and are unable to show accurately the early stages of enamel caries lesions.[36,37] Furthermore, this method is technique-sensitive and unavoidably exposes the patient to the hazards of ionizing radiation. Another factor is that radiographs do not indicate caries lesion activity and they are not able to detect the presence of cavitations (cavities), which is an important point in making a decision about treatment, mainly regarding proximal surfaces.[36] Nevertheless, the risk-benefit ratio of radiographic examination as an additional method for caries detection justifies its use and is now discussed in more detail.[37]

The bitewing method can aid the dentist in reaching an appropriate decision in both occlusal and proximal surfaces. In fact, in occlusal surfaces, if a tooth presents an ICDAS score of 0, 1, or 2, a radiograph is not necessary in most cases. If a site is classified as score 5 or 6 by visual inspection, a bitewing radiograph is not necessary to aid detection (periapical radiography can be indicated to check the proximity of the caries lesion to the pulp and to evaluate the condition of the periapical tissues). However, if the clinician scores the teeth as 3 or 4 in an occlusal site, a radiograph could be used to confirm the detection and to help in clinical decision making (nonsurgical or surgical treatment). Detection of caries lesions not detected by clinical examination, mainly early dentin caries lesions, favors the use of radiographic examination because the method has presented high sensitivity in detecting dentinal caries lesions.[36] Missed advanced dentin caries lesions could cause some discomfort for patients until the subsequent appointment, whereas nondetected enamel caries lesions do not pose any problem for the patient. Thus the radiographic method is beneficial, despite poor performance in detecting enamel caries lesions.

On occlusal surfaces, the radiographic method has been useful in detecting caries lesions not detected by visual inspection. These lesions have been termed hidden caries lesions.[38] However, it is mostly acknowledged that if a thorough clinical examination on cleaned and dried teeth has been done, "hidden" caries do not exist.[2,13,22]

For proximal surfaces, the benefits of radiographs are more evident. Teeth with an intact marginal ridge, and sound to visual examination, can have both enamel caries lesions and dentine caries lesions. In this instance, the presence of cavitation drives the decision to surgically restore rather than study the histologic lesion depth. In 1992, Pitts and Rimmer[39] correlated bitewing radiography with cavitation. Pitts and Rimmer demonstrated that when the radiographic image shows radiolucency restricted to the enamel, the caries lesion is usually noncavitated. Therefore, the dentist should opt for nonsurgical treatment if the lesion is active; for example, as judged by gingival status.[40] If the lesion reaches the internal half of dentin in the radiographic image, probably this lesion will present a cavitation.[39] Thus, surgical treatment is the best choice. However, when the radiographic image is an initial dentin caries lesion at the proximal surface, some caries lesions will present cavitation; but many of these surfaces will not have cavitation.[10] In these cases, therefore, the clinician could provide the temporary separation of the tooth with orthodontic rubbers, to check if the surface is cavitated[39] and determine the correct treatment decision. More common is the decision to plan for a new examination including a radiograph a year later, to monitor the progression and success of nonsurgical interventions.

Another possibility is digital radiography. In this technique, a digital sensor is used instead of conventional film and the radiographic image is stored in a computer. Digital radiographs usually expose patients to lower radiation doses than conventional methods. Digital radiographs permit the use of computer facilities, such as the possibilities of image enhancement and processing of the images, and of sending the images to other colleagues.[36,41] In general, conventional radiographic methods have presented sensitivity values around 0.50 to 0.60 and specificity values usually higher than 0.90 in detecting proximal caries lesions in primary and permanent teeth.[9,10,16,41]

For occlusal surfaces, the sensitivity values of conventional radiography have been between 0.50 and 0.80, and specificities around 0.80.[9,13,41,42] Digital methods have performed similarly.[36]

Novel tools, however, have been created for digital radiographic images to improve the process of caries detection or monitoring. Methods of digital subtraction can be used in 2 radiographic images of the same site recorded in different periods.[36,43] This method would allow for monitoring caries lesion progression,[43] because the 2 radiographs are taken with partly controlled projection angles.[36] Computed tomography techniques have been recommended for caries detection and seems a promising tool for this issue,[44] but further studies are necessary to check the performance and real benefits of the method.

In the use of the radiographic method as an adjunct of clinical examination in detecting caries, one can summarize that the conventional bitewing image can aid the dentist in reaching a treatment decision, mainly on proximal surfaces or occlusal sites scored as 3 or 4 by the ICDAS (see **Fig. 2**). Digital radiography has not presented a better performance, but the method exposes the patients to lower doses of ionizing radiation and could offer some assistance to the clinician.

Fiber Optic Transillumination

When a tooth is illuminated by a light, the carious tissue, because of the porosity, scatters the light and the enamel shows as a whiter, opaque area in visual inspection. Likewise, when the dentin is involved in the caries process, a shadow is observed in the underlying dentin. This phenomenon is observed in lesions classified as score 4 of the ICDAS.

The fiber optic transillumination (FOTI) method uses a high-intensity white light to enhance these effects. Thus, carious enamel and dentin appear as shadows with the use of the FOTI method.[45,46] The method is more appropriate for proximal surfaces but can be used for all surfaces. The device usually is portable and easy to use, but it is not quantitative and the diagnostic and treatment decisions depend on the dentist's interpretation. Therefore, low-reliability values are expected. A digital version of the technique, named digital fiber optic transillumination (DIFOTI), has been introduced, whereby the device records the images on a computer. These images can be archived and assessed in recalls.[46] This property could permit monitoring of surface demineralizations,[41] but this use of DIFOTI has not been tested as yet. One important property of DIFOTI is worth mentioning. Because the CCD camera takes an image of the surface only, it shows demineralization and does not correlate with cavitation; therefore, it should not be interpreted in the same manner as a bitewing radiograph.[47]

With regard to the performance of the FOTI method in detecting caries lesions, several studies have presented high specificities but low sensitivities for both occlusal and proximal surfaces.[9,41,45,46] The method does not use ionizing radiation. However, apart from this advantage, FOTI or DIFOTI methods have not presented more benefits than visual or radiographic methods.

Electronic Caries Monitor

The electronic caries monitor (ECM) device uses alternating current and measures the bulk resistance of tooth tissue.[46,48] The porosity of caries lesions is filled with fluids with high concentration of ions from the oral environment, and this more porous tissue decreases electrical resistance or impedance more than the sound dental tissue.[46] ECM is able to detect and quantify this difference.

The method presents a probe that is directly applied in an occlusal site, and the device shows a number that translates the electrical resistance of the site. Higher numbers indicate deeper caries lesions. As the method is quantitative, high-reproducibility values would be expected. Nevertheless, only fair reliability has been reported, probably due to technical problems. With regard to validity, higher sensitivity values (around 0.90) have been obtained compared with conventional methods, in detecting occlusal dentin caries lesions. However, lower specificity values (around 0.80) have been observed.[9,48] The decision about the activity status of the tooth should not be made using ECM alone, but the method could be useful as an adjunct to visual inspection. For use in daily clinical practice, however, the method has not presented advantages compared with conventional methods. Further, the method cannot yet be applied to proximal surfaces.

Fluorescence-Based Methods

The knowledge that the presence of a caries lesion provokes changes in the fluorescence properties of dental tissues has allowed the development of several fluorescence-based methods for detection and quantification of caries lesions. The first fluorescence-based method introduced onto the market was quantitative light-induced fluorescence (QLF). A QLF device uses a high-intensity halogen lamp, which emits a blue light ($\lambda = 370$ nm) to excite the tooth. When exposed to a light with this wavelength, dental tissues emit a fluorescence (in green spectrum), which is detected by the system, and the image is recorded in a computer. Mineral loss in this tooth causes a decrease in the fluorescence. This fluorescence reduction is analyzed by computer software and the mineral loss is quantified.[46,49]

The QLF method permits early detection of enamel demineralization (earlier than other methods). Furthermore, this method has presented a strong correlation with mineral loss of enamel caries lesions assessed by gold standard analytical methods (microradiography, for instance). Because of this property associated with high reliability values and a video repositioning software, which facilitates the acquisition of identical images on different occasions,[49] the device is an excellent method for monitoring enamel caries lesions to assess whether preventive measures are able to arrest or remineralize the lesion. Some clinical studies have used the QLF method to measure the effectiveness of preventive measures for initial caries lesions.[50] Nevertheless, the device is recommended more for smooth-surface caries lesions restricted to the enamel. The strong correlation with mineral content of the tooth decreases when the assessments are performed in dentin caries lesions.[49]

if the radiographic image indicates an initial dentin caries lesion (the outer third of dentin), the dentist should check for the presence of cavitation to decide which nonsurgical or surgical treatment is necessary. Here, temporary separation with orthodontic rubbers would be helpful. As an alternative for clinicians, Nyvad's system can be used instead of ICDAS.[6] Here, the treatment decision is made in a similar way to that described for ICDAS.

SUMMARY

Traditional thinking about caries management was not about diagnosis but about restoring the caries lesions. Current dental caries management considers caries disease to be a dynamic and reversible process.[6,63] The caries diagnosis process must take into account not only caries lesion detection but also the etiologic factors of dental caries and caries activity with regard to the disease and the lesions. Thus, the detection and assessment of caries lesions discussed in this article is only a part of the caries disease diagnosis process.

For caries lesion detection and assessment, visual inspection aided by a ball-ended probe is an essential method and must be performed in all patients. The use of indices, such as the ICDAS, improves the performance of the method mainly in terms of sensitivity and reliability. Through visual inspection the presence, severity, and activity of lesions must be assessed.

Other methods can be used as adjuncts to visual inspection. In the clinical practice setting, the most recommended additional method is radiography, using bitewing projection. Bitewing radiographs can aid the dentist in reaching a more appropriate treatment decision, mainly on proximal surfaces or occlusal caries lesions scored 3 or 4 on the ICDAS. New technologies have been developed and studied, but none has demonstrated significant benefits that justify use in daily clinical practice. For research purposes, however, new technologies could be useful. Further studies must be conducted to improve conventional methods, mainly in the assessment of caries lesion activity. Studies must also be conducted to find a new technology with better performance than conventional methods, or a new method that permits a more objective assessment of caries lesion activity.

The ICDAS, including the activity assessment system or the Nyvad system, seems to be the best option for a final caries diagnosis.

REFERENCES

1. Thylstrup A, Fejerskov O. Textbook of clinical cariology. 2nd edition. Copenhagen (Denmark): Munksgaard; 1994.
2. Ekstrand KR, Ricketts DN, Kidd EA. Occlusal caries: pathology, diagnosis and logical management. Dent Update 2001;28(8):380–7.
3. Bader JD, Shugars DA. What do we know about how dentists make caries-related treatment decisions? Community Dent Oral Epidemiol 1997;25(1):97–103.
4. Nyvad B, Fejerskov O. Assessing the stage of caries lesion activity on the basis of clinical and microbiological examination. Community Dent Oral Epidemiol 1997; 25(1):69–75.
5. Basting RT, Serra MC. Occlusal caries: diagnosis and noninvasive treatments. Quintessence Int 1999;30(3):174–8.
6. Nyvad B. Diagnosis versus detection of caries. Caries Res 2004;38(3):192–8.
7. Baelum V, Heidmann J, Nyvad B. Dental caries paradigms in diagnosis and diagnostic research. Eur J Oral Sci 2006;114(4):263–77.

8. Pitts NB. Current methods and criteria for caries diagnosis in Europe. J Dent Educ 1993;57(6):409–14.
9. Bader JD, Shugars DA, Bonito AJ. A systematic review of the performance of methods for identifying carious lesions. J Public Health Dent 2002;62(4): 201–13.
10. Braga MM, Morais CC, Nakama RC, et al. In vitro performance of methods of approximal caries detection in primary molars. Oral Surg Oral Med Oral Pathol Oral Radiol Endod 2009;108(4):e35–41.
11. Ekstrand KR. Improving clinical visual detection—potential for caries clinical trials. J Dent Res 2004;83(Spec Issue, No C):C67–71.
12. Ekstrand KR, Kuzmina I, Bjorndal L, et al. Relationship between external and histologic features of progressive stages of caries in the occlusal fossa. Caries Res 1995;29(4):243–50.
13. Ekstrand KR, Ricketts DN, Kidd EA. Reproducibility and accuracy of three methods for assessment of demineralization depth of the occlusal surface: an in vitro examination. Caries Res 1997;31(3):224–31.
14. Nyvad B, Machiulskiene V, Baelum V. Reliability of a new caries diagnostic system differentiating between active and inactive caries lesions. Caries Res 1999;33(4):252–60.
15. Braga MM, Mendes FM, Martignon S, et al. In vitro Comparison of Nyvad's system and ICDAS-II with lesion activity assessment for evaluation of severity and activity of occlusal caries lesions in primary teeth. Caries Res 2009;43(5):405–12.
16. Novaes TF, Matos R, Braga MM, et al. Performance of a pen-type laser fluorescence device and conventional methods in detecting approximal caries lesions in primary teeth—in vivo study. Caries Res 2009;43(1):36–42.
17. Braga MM, Oliveira LB, Bonini GA, et al. Feasibility of the International Caries Detection and Assessment System (ICDAS-II) in epidemiological surveys and comparability with standard World Health Organization criteria. Caries Res 2009;43(4):245–9.
18. Ismail AI. Visual and visuo-tactile detection of dental caries. J Dent Res 2004; 83(Spec Issue, No C):C56–66.
19. Ekstrand K, Qvist V, Thylstrup A. Light microscope study of the effect of probing in occlusal surfaces. Caries Res 1987;21(4):368–74.
20. Kuhnisch J, Dietz W, Stosser L, et al. Effects of dental probing on occlusal surfaces—a scanning electron microscopy evaluation. Caries Res 2007;41(1): 43–8.
21. Pitts N. "ICDAS"—an international system for caries detection and assessment being developed to facilitate caries epidemiology, research and appropriate clinical management. Community Dent Health 2004;21(3):193–8.
22. Ekstrand KR, Ricketts DN, Kidd EA, et al. Detection, diagnosing, monitoring and logical treatment of occlusal caries in relation to lesion activity and severity: an in vivo examination with histological validation. Caries Res 1998;32(4):247–54.
23. Ismail AI, Sohn W, Tellez M, et al. The International Caries Detection and Assessment System (ICDAS): an integrated system for measuring dental caries. Community Dent Oral Epidemiol 2007;35(3):170–8.
24. Ekstrand KR, Martignon S, Ricketts DJ, et al. Detection and activity assessment of primary coronal caries lesions: a methodologic study. Oper Dent 2007;32(3): 225–35.
25. Jablonski-Momeni A, Stachniss V, Ricketts DN, et al. Reproducibility and accuracy of the ICDAS-II for detection of occlusal caries in vitro. Caries Res 2008; 42(2):79–87.

26. Rodrigues JA, Hug I, Diniz MB, et al. Performance of fluorescence methods, radiographic examination and ICDAS II on occlusal surfaces in vitro. Caries Res 2008;42(4):297–304.
27. Shoaib L, Deery C, Ricketts DN, et al. Validity and Reproducibility of ICDAS II in Primary Teeth. Caries Res 2009;43(6):442–8.
28. Mortimer KV. The relationship of deciduous enamel structure to dental disease. Caries Res 1970;4(3):206–23.
29. Shellis RP. Relationship between human enamel structure and the formation of caries-like lesions in vitro. Arch Oral Biol 1984;29(12):975–81.
30. Kuhnisch J, Berger S, Goddon I, et al. Occlusal caries detection in permanent molars according to WHO basic methods, ICDAS II and laser fluorescence measurements. Community Dent Oral Epidemiol 2008;36(6):475–84.
31. Varma S, Banerjee A, Bartlett D. An in vivo investigation of associations between saliva properties, caries prevalence and potential lesion activity in an adult UK population. J Dent 2008;36(4):294–9.
32. Ekstrand KR, Zero DT, Martignon S, et al. Lesion activity assessment. Monogr Oral Sci 2009;21:63–90.
33. Baelum V, Machiulskiene V, Nyvad B, et al. Application of survival analysis to carious lesion transitions in intervention trials. Community Dent Oral Epidemiol 2003;31(4):252–60.
34. Mialhe FL, Pereira AC, Pardi V, et al. Comparison of three methods for detection of carious lesions in proximal surfaces versus direct visual examination after tooth separation. J Clin Pediatr Dent 2003;28(1):59–62.
35. Peers A, Hill FJ, Mitropoulos CM, et al. Validity and reproducibility of clinical examination, fibre-optic transillumination, and bite-wing radiology for the diagnosis of small approximal carious lesions: an in vitro study. Caries Res 1993;27(4):307–11.
36. Wenzel A. Bitewing and digital bitewing radiography for detection of caries lesions. J Dent Res 2004;83(Spec Issue, No C):C72–5.
37. Pitts NB. The use of bitewing radiographs in the management of dental caries: scientific and practical considerations. Dentomaxillofac Radiol 1996;25(1):5–16.
38. Weerheijm KL. Occlusal 'hidden caries'. Dental Update 1997;24(5):182–4.
39. Pitts NB, Rimmer PA. An in vivo comparison of radiographic and directly assessed clinical caries status of posterior approximal surfaces in primary and permanent teeth. Caries Res 1992;26(2):146–52.
40. Ekstrand KR, Bruun G, Bruun M. Plaque and gingival status as indicators for caries progression on approximal surfaces. Caries Res 1998;32(1):41–5.
41. Yang J, Dutra V. Utility of radiology, laser fluorescence, and transillumination. Dent Clin North Am 2005;49(4):739–52.
42. Mendes FM, Ganzerla E, Nunes AF, et al. Use of high-powered magnification to detect occlusal caries in primary teeth. Am J Dent 2006;19(1):19–22.
43. Ricketts DN, Ekstrand KR, Martignon S, et al. Accuracy and reproducibility of conventional radiographic assessment and subtraction radiography in detecting demineralization in occlusal surfaces. Caries Res 2007;41(2):121–8.
44. Tyndall DA, Rathore S. Cone-beam CT diagnostic applications: caries, periodontal bone assessment, and endodontic applications. Dent Clin North Am 2008;52(4):825–41.
45. Cortes DF, Ellwood RP, Ekstrand KR. An in vitro comparison of a combined FOTI/visual examination of occlusal caries with other caries diagnostic methods and the effect of stain on their diagnostic performance. Caries Res 2003;37(1):8–16.
46. Pretty IA. Caries detection and diagnosis: novel technologies. J Dent 2006;34(10):727–39.

47. Young DA, Featherstone JD. Digital imaging fiber-optic trans-illumination, F-speed radiographic film and depth of approximal lesions. J Am Dent Assoc 2005;136(12):1682–7.
48. Longbottom C, Huysmans MC. Electrical measurements for use in caries clinical trials. J Dent Res 2004;83(Spec Issue, No C):C76–9.
49. Angmar-Mansson B, ten Bosch JJ. Quantitative light-induced fluorescence (QLF): a method for assessment of incipient caries lesions. Dentomaxillofac Radiol 2001;30(6):298–307.
50. Al-Khateeb S, Forsberg CM, de Josselin de Jong E, et al. A longitudinal laser fluorescence study of white spot lesions in orthodontic patients. Am J Orthod Dentofacial Orthop 1998;113(6):595–602.
51. Kuhnisch J, Ifland S, Tranaeus S, et al. In vivo detection of non-cavitated caries lesions on occlusal surfaces by visual inspection and quantitative light-induced fluorescence. Acta Odontol Scand 2007;65(3):183–8.
52. Stookey GK. Quantitative light fluorescence: a technology for early monitoring of the caries process. Dent Clin North Am 2005;49(4):753–70.
53. Hibst R, Paulus R, Lussi A. Detection of occlusal caries by laser fluorescence: basic and clinical investigations. Med Laser Appl 2001;16:205–13.
54. Mendes FM, de Oliveira E, Araujo de Faria DL, et al. Ability of laser fluorescence device associated with fluorescent dyes in detecting and quantifying early smooth surface caries lesions. J Biomed Opt 2006;11(2):24007.
55. Mendes FM, Hissadomi M, Imparato JC. Effects of drying time and the presence of plaque on the in vitro performance of laser fluorescence in occlusal caries of primary teeth. Caries Res 2004;38(2):104–8.
56. Mendes FM, Nicolau J. Utilization of laser fluorescence to monitor caries lesions development in primary teeth. J Dent Child 2004;71(2):139–42.
57. Bengtson AL, Gomes AC, Mendes FM, et al. Influence of examiner's clinical experience in detecting occlusal caries lesions in primary teeth. Pediatr Dent 2005;27(3):238–43.
58. Braga MM, Mendes FM, Imparato JC, et al. Effect of cut-off points on performance of laser fluorescence for detecting occlusal caries. J Clin Pediatr Dent 2007;32(1):33–6.
59. Lussi A, Megert B, Longbottom C, et al. Clinical performance of a laser fluorescence device for detection of occlusal caries lesions. Eur J Oral Sci 2001;109(1):14–9.
60. Lussi A, Longbottom C, Gygax M, et al. Influence of professional cleaning and drying of occlusal surfaces on laser fluorescence in vivo. Caries Res 2005;39(4):284–6.
61. Lussi A, Reich E. The influence of toothpastes and prophylaxis pastes on fluorescence measurements for caries detection in vitro. Eur J Oral Sci 2005;113(2):141–4.
62. Bader JD, Shugars DA. A systematic review of the performance of a laser fluorescence device for detecting caries. J Am Dent Assoc 2004;135(10):1413–26.
63. Lussi A, Hack A, Hug I, et al. Detection of approximal caries with a new laser fluorescence device. Caries Res 2006;40(2):97–103.

Implementing Caries Risk Assessment and Clinical Interventions

Douglas A. Young, DDS, MS, MBA[a],
John D.B. Featherstone, MSc, PhD[b],*

KEYWORDS

- Caries management by risk assessment
- Caries risk assessment • Caries-protective factors
- Caries disease

Caries management by risk assessment (CAMBRA) is an evidence-based approach to preventing, reversing and, when necessary, repairing early damage to teeth.[1,2] Unlike the classic medical model of "one pathogen—one disease," the CAMBRA model is built on the understanding that dental caries is a disease initiated by a complex biofilm (rather than one pathogen) which changes dynamically with its environment (tooth, pellicle, saliva). Thus, rather than focusing on the elimination of one pathogen, CAMBRA must determine which of many factors is causing the expression of disease and take corrective action.

THE CARIES BALANCE/IMBALANCE MODEL

The caries balance/imbalance model is a visual representation of the multifactorial nature of the disease known as dental caries. The model is a reminder of the determining factors of caries disease and illustrates the dynamic interaction of the biofilm with the oral environment. It is the environment that determines how the biofilm will behave and whether the disease is severe enough to demineralize the teeth and cause visible changes. By applying actual patient information to the caries balance, an astute clinician can "assess" the risk of future demineralization based on weighing all the disease indicators and risk factors against existing protective factors. This process is called a caries risk assessment (CRA).

[a] Department of Dental Practice, University of the Pacific, Arthur A. Dugoni School of Dentistry, 2155 Webster Street, Suite 400, San Francisco, CA 94115, USA
[b] University of California San Francisco, School of Dentistry, 513 Parnassus Avenue, Box 0430, San Francisco, CA 94143-0430, USA
* Corresponding author.
E-mail address: jdbf@ucsf.edu

Dent Clin N Am 54 (2010) 495–505
doi:10.1016/j.cden.2010.04.002
0011-8532/10/$ – see front matter © 2010 Elsevier Inc. All rights reserved.

CARIES RISK FACTORS

Caries risk factors are biologic factors that contribute to the level of risk for the patient of having new caries lesions in the future or having the existing lesions progress (see **Table 1**). The risk factors are the biologic factors that have contributed to the disease or will contribute to the future manifestation of the disease on the tooth. These pathologic factors not only tell us what is out of balance but also suggest how the imbalance can be corrected. **Fig. 1** lists only the 3 risk factors that research has proven to be "causative" of caries lesions (given a pathogenic environment) and can be easily remembered because their first letters spell the word "BAD":

Bad bacteria (meaning cariogenic bacteria),
Absence of saliva (hyposalivation),
Dietary habits that are poor (frequent ingestion of fermentable carbohydrates).

The CRA form shown in **Table 1** lists several other risk factors (totaling 9) identified as outcomes measures of CRA[4]: (1) medium or high MS (mutans streptococci) and LB (*Lactobacillus* species) counts, (2) visible heavy plaque on teeth, (3) frequent (>3 times daily) snacking between meals, (4) deep pits and fissures, (5) recreational drug use, (6) inadequate saliva flow by observation or measurement, (7) saliva-reducing factors (medications/radiation/systemic), (8) exposed roots, and (9) orthodontic appliances.

CARIES-PROTECTIVE FACTORS

Caries-protective factors are biologic or therapeutic factors that can collectively offset the pathologic challenge presented by the aforementioned caries risk factors (see **Table 1**). The more severe the caries risk factors, the higher the intensity of protective factors must be to keep the patient in balance or to reverse the caries process. **Fig. 1** only lists a few that are known to be highly protective and can be remembered by the acronym "SAFE":

Saliva and sealants,
Antibacterials,
Fluoride, and
Effective dietary habits.

Industry is responding to the need for more and better products to treat dental caries disease, and the current list in **Table 1** is sure to expand in the near future. At present, the protective factors listed in **Table 1** are: (1) lives/work/school located in a fluoridated community, (2) fluoride toothpaste at least once daily, (3) fluoride toothpaste at least twice daily, (4) fluoride mouth rinse (0.05% NaF) daily, (5) 5000 ppm F fluoride toothpaste daily, (6) fluoride varnish in last 6 months, (7) office fluoride topical in last 6 months, (8) chlorhexidine prescribed/used daily for 1 week each of the last 6 months, (9) xylitol gum/lozenges 4 times daily in the last 6 months, (10) calcium and phosphate supplement paste during the last 6 months, and (11) adequate saliva flow (>1 mL/min stimulated). Fluoride toothpaste frequency is included because studies have shown that brushing twice daily or more is significantly more effective than brushing once a day or less.[6] Any or all of these protective factors can contribute to keep the patient "in balance" and to enhance remineralization, which is the natural repair process of the early carious lesion.

CARIES RISK ASSESSMENT

A CRA is simply a way to gather the "evidence" in the most predicable fashion to diagnose current caries disease, help predict future disease, and to determine what factors are out of balance so evidence-based clinical decisions can be made.[7–9] The CRA may draw on relevant historical data of the patient such as medical history (medications, acid reflux), dental history (previous caries experience), social history (drugs, alcohol, smoking), dietary history, and any other personal or cultural habits that could contribute to caries disease. Lastly, a CRA may also rely on additional tests such as saliva/pH assessment and bacterial load assessment.

Implementation of a CRA in clinical practice is best done by the use of a CRA form. This form ensures that each patient will be systematically assessed in the same manner based on the best available research. The CRA form presented here is based on published science and outcomes measures of the use of the form. The items in the form have been trimmed to include only those that had significant relationships to the onset of future cavitation in thousands of patients. The aim is to keep the form and procedure as simple and rapid as possible for use in practice, to limit it to one page, and to have only proven components included. The CRA form presented here is based on the caries balance/imbalance theory, and the factors evaluated were discussed previously. Although there are several published CRA forms, the one shown in **Table 1** was chosen to use as an example in this article because the content of the form and the procedures have been validated by published results of research using a large cohort of patients.[4] The included items all had statistically significant odds ratios relating to the future onset of cavitation. This form and a CRA form for children younger than 6 years (as well as other useful articles that may help in CAMBRA implementation) can be downloaded from the following Web site—www.cdafoundation. org/journal—by selecting the October and November 2007 CDA journals.

To use the form (see **Table 1**) one simply circles the yes answers, counts them, and visualizes how these will affect the balance at the bottom of the form. The practitioner will thus be able to readily determine low, moderate, high, or extreme risk. Extreme risk is high risk plus major salivary dysfunction (hyposalivation). Low risk should indicate that there is a very low risk of future dental caries disease, provided no deleterious changes are made. On the other hand, high risk indicates the high likelihood of new caries lesions in the near future (a year or two). If there is doubt about low or high risk, then the classification is moderate.

There are several other versions of CRA forms available, and clinical outcomes of using many risk indicators and factors are summarized in a systematic review by Zero and colleagues.[8] In addition, there are differences in the relative predictive value given to different factors in the literature (eg, according to the 2001 NIH Consensus Conference on Dental Caries, presence of mutans streptococci alone is no more than weakly predictive of clinical caries activity).[9] However, none of these other forms have published outcomes results. The American Dental Association offers caries assessment forms for patients 0 to 6 years old, and those older than 6 years. The forms can be found here: http://www.ada.org/sections/newsAndEvents/docs/ topics_caries_instructions.pdf. In addition, the American Academy of Pediatric Dentistry also offers their form for children younger than 6 years at: http://www. aapd.org/media/Policies_Guidelines/P_CariesRiskAssess.pdf.

All these forms vary from each other in some way or another; however, all of them agree that caries experience is the strongest predictor of future caries disease, even though they may use different variables to describe caries experience. In addition, they all measure the other etiologic factors involved in the disease in some manner; the weight

Table 2
Caries management by risk assessment: clinical guidelines for patients 6 years and older

Risk Level[c,d]	Frequency of Radiographs	Frequency of Caries Recall Examinations	Saliva Test (Saliva Flow & Bacterial Culture)	Antimicrobials Chlorhexidine Xylitol	Fluoride	pH Control	Calcium Phosphate Topical Supplements	Sealants (Resin-based or Glass Ionomer)
Low risk	Bitewing radiographs every 24–36 mo	Every 6–12 mo to reevaluate caries risk	May be done as a baseline reference for new patients	Per saliva test if done	OTC fluoride-containing toothpaste twice daily, after breakfast and at bedtime. Optional: NaF varnish if excessive root exposure or sensitivity	Not required	Not required Optional: for excessive root exposure or sensitivity	Optional
Moderate risk	Bitewing radiographs every 18–24 mo	Every 4–6 mo to reevaluate caries risk	May be done as a baseline reference for new patients or if there is suspicion of high bacterial challenge and to assess efficacy and patient cooperation	Per saliva test if done Xylitol (6–10 g/d) gum or candies. Two tabs of gum or 2 candies 4 times daily	OTC fluoride-containing toothpaste twice daily plus 0.05% NaF rinse daily Initially, 1–2 applications of NaF varnish; 1 application at 4–6 mo recall	Not required	Not required Optional: for excessive root exposure or sensitivity	As per ICDAS Sealant Protocol

	Bitewing radiographs		Saliva flow test and bacterial culture	Chlorhexidine	1.1% NaF toothpaste		Calcium/phosphate paste	Sealants
High risk[a]	Bitewing radiographs every 6–18 mo or until no cavitated lesions are evident	Every 3–4 mo to reevaluate caries risk and apply fluoride varnish	Saliva flow test and bacterial culture initially and at every caries recall appointment to assess efficacy and patient cooperation	Chlorhexidine gluconate 0.12% 10-mL rinse for 1 min daily for 1 wk each mo. Xylitol (6–10 g/d) gum or candies. Two tabs of gum or 2 candies 4 times daily	1.1% NaF toothpaste twice daily instead of regular fluoride toothpaste. Initially, 1–3 applications of NaF varnish; 1 application at 3–4 mo recall	Not required	Optional. Apply calcium/phosphate paste several times daily	As per ICDAS Sealant Protocol
Extreme risk[b] (high risk plus dry mouth)	Bitewing radiographs every 6 mo or until no cavitated lesions are evident	Every 3 mo to reevaluate caries risk and apply fluoride varnish	Saliva flow test and bacterial culture initially and at every caries recall appointment to assess efficacy and patient cooperation	Chlorhexidine 0.12% (preferably CHX in water base rinse) 10-mL rinse for 1 min daily for 1 wk each mo. Xylitol (6–10 g/d) gum or candies. Two tabs of gum or 2 candies 4 times daily	1.1% NaF toothpaste twice daily instead of regular fluoride toothpaste. Initially, 1–3 applications NaF varnish; 1 application at 3 mo recall	Acid neutralizing rinses as needed if mouth feels dry, after snacking, bedtime and after breakfast Baking soda gum as needed	Required. Apply calcium/phosphate paste twice daily	As per ICDAS Sealant Protocol

[a] Patients with one (or more) cavitated lesion(s) are high-risk patients.

[b] Patients with one (or more) cavitated lesion(s) and severe xerostomia are extreme-risk patients.

[c] All restorative work to be done with the minimally invasive philosophy in mind. Existing smooth surface lesions that do not penetrate the DEJ and are not cavitated should be treated chemically not surgically. For extreme-risk patients use holding care with glass ionomer materials until caries progression is controlled. Patients with appliances (RPDs, Orthodontics) require excellent oral hygiene together with intensive fluoride therapy (eg, high fluoride toothpaste and fluoride varnish every 3 months). Where indicated, antimicrobial therapy is to be done in conjunction with restorative work.

[d] For all risk levels: Patients must maintain good oral hygiene and a diet low in frequency of fermentable carbohydrates.

From Jenson L, Budenz AW, Featherstone JD, et al. Clinical protocols for caries management by risk assessment. J Calif Dent Assoc 2007;35(10):714–23; with permission.

that these other factors receive varies from form to form, in part because the literature on risk assessment (except for past caries experience)is very limited and scarce.

Any CRA form should systematically "weigh" the factors that research has proven to be pathogenic against the protective factors that are known to protect from caries disease. The astute clinician can then manipulate these environmental factors via treatment interventions that will tip the caries balance to favor health. Because not all factors have equal predictive value, the questions used in any CRA form must be "weighted" in some fashion. The weighting system shown in **Table 1** is a visual weighting system created by the 3-column format based on outcomes research and statistical odds ratios mentioned previously. Other forms may use a mathematical weighting system.

The result of any CRA is to combine historical data, information from the CRA form, including any additional test such as saliva or pH assessment and bacterial load assessment, to ultimately allow a determination of an overall caries risk for the patient. This will help establish a caries disease diagnosis and disease activity level (caries active or caries inactive). Caries risk changes with time and needs to be reassessed as time goes on.

CLINICAL INTERVENTION PROTOCOLS

Once overall caries risk (low, moderate, high, or extreme) is determined, there must be therapeutic intervention protocols attached to the risk level for that patient so that treatment options along with prognosis can be presented to the patient and a treatment plan formulated. This process is CAMBRA, whereby the level and type of risk is used to determine the level and type of corrective therapeutic intervention. The problem is that there currently is no one correct treatment protocol, just as there is no one correct way to assess the caries risk of the patient. Randomized clinical trials and systematic reviews will always be lacking where clinical practice dictates that multiple treatment interventions must be employed to treat a complex multifactorial disease. That said, a table with a suggested protocol as an example of what interventions could be done based on the caries risk level of the patient is included here. Other articles in this issue look at the levels of evidence supporting the use of therapeutic interventions in much greater detail. **Table 2** presents an example protocol published for age 6 to adult based on caries risk category,[10] and can be obtained in the October 2007 CDA journal at www.cdafoundation.org/journal. The 8 interventions summarized in **Table 2** are: (1) frequency of radiographs, (2) frequency of caries recall examinations, (3) saliva test (flow and bacterial culture), (4) antibacterials, (5) fluoride, (6) pH control, (7) calcium phosphate topical supplements, and (8) sealants (resin-based or glass ionomer).

Individualized, evidence-based treatment options along with prognosis is presented to the patient, and decisions are made based on the patient's current risk data along with clinical experience and patient input. Implementation of the treatment phase requires the clinician to assist the patient in modification of behaviors that favor health; this will require skill in obtaining patient cooperation in the use of recommended therapeutic interventions. In doing so it is important to give patients encouragement and clear instructions on what they need to do. Appendix 1 gives examples of patient instruction letters for each risk category.

SUMMARY

Dental caries is a complex multifactorial disease that cannot be controlled by restoration alone. A CRA is a way to systematically measure which factors are out of balance and which will cause demineralization, as well as the risk of future disease in a given patient. To assist the clinician in assessing caries risk, several forms and procedures are in existence, of which one form and one example protocol is used in this article to illustrate how CAMBRA can be conducted in clinical practice. Other articles in this issue evaluate the levels of evidence of many of these suggested interventions.

APPENDIX 1: SAMPLE PATIENT LETTERS/RECOMMENDATIONS FOR CONTROL OF DENTAL DECAY (AGES 6 AND OVER/ADULT)

One of the following letters including home care recommendations should go to each patient depending on the risk category and the overall treatment plan.

LOW CARIES RISK

Dear …………..(patient's name),
  Congratulations, according to your examination findings, you are at low risk for future dental decay.
  Please continue doing the following:

- Brush twice daily with fluoride-containing toothpaste.
- Keep up with your current healthy dietary habits and avoid frequent carbohydrate (sugary) snacks and drinks.
- The follow-up appointments will be set up to monitor your oral healthy every year.

MODERATE CARIES RISK

Dear ……………(patient's name),
  According to your examination findings, you are at *moderate risk* for developing new cavities in the future.
  To reduce the risk, please do the following:

- Brush twice daily with prescription fluoride toothpaste (Control Rx or Prevident 5000 Plus) instead of your regular toothpaste.
- Chew or suck xylitol-containing gum or candies: 2 pieces 3 to 4 times daily.
- Reduce the number of carbohydrate-rich snacks between meals, including candies, mints, cookies, juice, soda, etc. It is better to snack food rich in protein, such as cheese and nuts rather than starch/sugar.
- We will reevaluate your risk every 6 months.

HIGH CARIES RISK

Dear ………………..(patient's name),
  The results of your examination indicate that you are at *high risk* for development of new cavities in the near future.
  To reduce the risk, please do the following:

PRESCRIPTION TOOTHPASTE
  Brush twice daily with either Control Rx or Prevident 5000 Plus instead of your regular toothpaste.

PRESCRIPTION MOUTH RINSE
  Peridex or PerioGard. Use for 1 week each month: rinse once a day (at bedtime) with 10 mL for 1 minute, at least 1 hour after using the 5000 ppm F toothpaste.

REDUCE SNACKS
Reduce the number of carbohydrate-rich snacks between meals, including candies, mints, cookies, juices, sodas, etc. It is better to snack food rich in protein, such as cheese and nuts rather than starch/sugar.

XYLITOL
We recommend that you suck or chew xylitol mints or gum 2 pieces 3 to 4 times daily.

MI Paste: Plus
Use in the morning and at night, after brushing with fluoride toothpaste. Apply a pea-size amount of MI paste to tooth surface using a finger. Leave undisturbed for 3 minutes. Do not rinse. It is safe to swallow the paste.

Continuation of caries (cavity) control regime (re-examinations done every 3 months):

- Assessment of your risk for future cavity development; review of oral hygiene.
- Test cavity causing bacteria levels in saliva to evaluate effect of the preventive treatment.
- Apply fluoride varnish to strengthen your teeth.

We will provide you with a timetable to help you to remember all of these procedures.

Further follow-up treatment: We will continue to monitor your progress at appropriate time intervals.

EXTREME CARIES RISK (HIGH RISK PLUS SEVERE SALIVARY GLAND HYPOFUNCTION)

Dear ....(patient's name),
The results of your examination indicate that you are at *extreme risk* for development of new cavities in the near future.
To reduce the risk, please do the following:

PRESCRIPTION TOOTHPASTE
Brush twice daily with either Control Rx or Prevident 5000 Plus instead of your regular toothpaste.

PRESCRIPTION MOUTH RINSE
Peridex or PerioGard. Use for 1 week each month : rinse once a day (at bedtime) with 10 mL, for 1 minute, at least 1 hour after using the 5000 ppm F toothpaste

BAKING SODA RINSE
Use a baking soda rinse 4 to 6 times daily during the day, ie, after each meal or snack. (The rinse is made by mixing 2 teaspoons of baking soda in an 8-oz bottle of water)

REDUCE SNACKS
Reduce the number of carbohydrate-rich snacks between meals, including candies, mints, cookies, juices, sodas, etc. It is better to snack on food rich in protein, such as cheese and nuts rather than starch/sugar.

XYLITOL
We recommend that you suck or chew xylitol mints or gum 2 pieces 3 to 4 times daily.

MI Paste: Plus
> Use in the morning and at night, after brushing with fluoride toothpaste. Apply a pea-size amount of MI paste to tooth surface using a finger. Leave undisturbed for 3 minutes. Do not rinse. It is safe to swallow the paste.

Continuation of caries (cavity) control regime (re-examinations done every 3 months):

- Assessment of your risk for future cavity development; review of oral hygiene.
- Test cavity causing bacteria levels in saliva to evaluate effect of the preventive treatment.
- Apply fluoride varnish to strengthen your teeth.

We will provide you with a timetable to help you to remember all of these procedures.

Further follow-up treatment: We will continue to monitor your progress at appropriate time intervals.

REFERENCES

1. Young DA, Featherstone JD, Roth JR. Curing the silent epidemic: caries management in the 21st century and beyond. J Calif Dent Assoc 2007;35(10):681–5.
2. Featherstone JD, Domejean-Orliaguet S, Jenson L, et al. Caries risk assessment in practice for age 6 through adult. J Calif Dent Assoc 2007;35(10):703–7.
3. Featherstone JD. The caries balance: contributing factors and early detection. J Calif Dent Assoc 2003;31(2):129–33.
4. Domejean-Orliaguet S, Gansky SA, Featherstone JD. Caries risk assessment in an educational environment. J Dent Educ 2006;70(12):1346–54.
5. Featherstone JDB, Gansky SA, Hoover CI, et al. A randomized clinical trial of caries management by risk assessment [abstract #25]. Caries Res 2005;39:295.
6. Curnow MM, Pine CM, Burnside G, et al. A randomised controlled trial of the efficacy of supervised toothbrushing in high-caries-risk children. Caries Res 2002; 36(4):294–300.
7. Featherstone JD. The caries balance: the basis for caries management by risk assessment. Oral Health Prev Dent 2004;2(Suppl 1):259–64.
8. Zero D, Fontana M, Lennon AM. Clinical applications and outcomes of using indicators of risk in caries management. J Dent Educ 2001;65(10):1126–32.
9. National Institutes of Health. Diagnosis and management of dental caries throughout life. Consensus Development Conference statement, March 26–28, 2001. J Dent Educ 2001;65:1162–8.
10. Jenson L, Budenz AW, Featherstone JD, et al. Clinical protocols for caries management by risk assessment. J Calif Dent Assoc 2007;35(10):714–23.

Strategies for Noninvasive Demineralized Tissue Repair

Mathilde C. Peters, DMD, PhD

KEYWORDS

- Tissue repair • Remineralization • Fluoride
- Calcium-based strategies • Sealants • Infiltration • Lasers

Traditional management of a caries lesion primarily was focused on operative treatment. This often started an irreversible, restorative cycle, leading to several replacements over time with increasing restoration size and every so often iatrogenic damage. The last two decades have seen a growing insight about the process of lesion development and its causal and continual factors. This awareness changed the paradigm of Black's "extension for prevention" into the motto "extension of prevention".[1] The effect of caries disease in the tissue sets off/prompts lesion formation. Once the first clinically visible signs have been discovered, the detection should be followed by diagnosis of severity and extent of the lesion and whether it is an active process or not. Presence of tissue damage alone is not sufficient for management decisions as the present lesion might be rather a scar than a sign of current activity.

Fortunately, recognition of caries as a multifactorial disease process involving the biofilm has received more and more attention. The first step in contemporary caries management is focused on the various options to cope with the locally out-of-balance oral biofilm and stop progression of the disease (see the articles by Philip D. Marsh; and Svante Twetman elsewhere in this issue for further exploration of this topic). After the caries process has been halted, causative factors need to be evaluated and individual treatment regimens installed that will prevent new occurrence of the caries disease. Caries lesions develop by dissolution of minerals from the tooth tissues, leaving behind a more porous structure. Therapies that focus on rebalancing the interplay between demineralization and remineralization (see the article by Young and Featherstone elsewhere in this issue for further exploration of this topic), tipping the balance toward an overriding mineral uptake in the tissue, not only result in repair of the damage done, but concurrently assist in preventing new lesions of forming.

Department of Cariology, Restorative Sciences and Endodontics, School of Dentistry, University of Michigan, 1011 North University Avenue, Ann Arbor, MI 48109-1078, USA
E-mail address: mcpete@umich.edu

Dent Clin N Am 54 (2010) 507–525
doi:10.1016/j.cden.2010.03.005
0011-8532/10/$ – see front matter © 2010 Elsevier Inc. All rights reserved.

This article focuses on the repair of affected hard tooth tissues using noninvasive management strategies. Such an approach takes into account the dynamic nature of the caries disease process (see the article by Hara and Zero elsewhere in this issue for further exploration of this topic). For successful noninvasive management, the lesions have to be detected early on, so they can be managed in a nonoperative way.[2] This type of early caries management requires special clinical attention, detection, and diagnostic skills (see the article by Braga and colleagues elsewhere in this issue for further exploration of this topic). It is time-consuming, but reestablishing the integrity of the tooth surface early on in the caries process will bring great rewards for patients. Their tooth structures will be preserved, and costly, extensive restorative treatments in the future prevented.

THE DISEASE—A SLOW-PACED PROCESS

The equilibrium that exists between plaque fluids and apatite crystals at the tooth surface is constantly overwhelmed by pH fluctuations at the plaque–tooth interface. In a healthy mouth, this is a normal physiologic process that takes place at a subclinical level numerous times a day. During periods of neutral pH, lost minerals are replaced by calcium and phosphates from saliva, forming a hard outer surface. A continual ion exchange, in both directions across the tooth surface interface, attempts to reestablish the mineral balance. The caries lesion is a result of loss of mineral from the dental tissues. Caries is not a disease process that develops rapidly, but it takes time for the effect (ie, lesion) to develop. Initial lesions undergo a constant daily battle between progression and regression. It may take 3 to 4 years to develop a cavitation.[3] Not all initial lesions, however, develop to cavities at the same rate.[4] The progression rates are not the same for each site,[5] and they are independent of the patient's decayed, missing or filled surfaces (DMFS).[3]

In general, there is ample time—between lesion initiation in enamel and subsequent progression into dentin involvement—to interrupt this process using preventive and repair strategies. Preventive management strategies can effectively arrest and even completely reverse the caries process. It is therefore important to detect lesions in their early stage. Reasons for slower pace of lesion progression in the last three decades are not clearly defined, but increased use of fluoride may have attributed to lower progression rates of fissure caries for example. Some lesions may have become arrested. This will lead to clinically undetected carious dentin at the base of occlusal fissures. This phenomenon, reported since 1931,[6] received renewed attention in the 1990s.[7,8] When initial lesions are taken into account, however, the percentage of clinically undetected carious dentin lesions dropped dramatically to less than 2%[9] and were in the same order of magnitude as pre-eruptive lesions.[10]

A critical period for rapid caries development occurs when a tooth erupts in the oral environment and the enamel is not yet fully matured. Continuous exposure to saliva promotes full maturation. This maturation and the continuing demineralization/remineralization processes lead to a more acid-resistant outer enamel. The time during eruption and immediately after is the most vulnerable period for caries development. Caries initiation and progression rates of permanent molars are highest during this early posteruptive period.[11] Additional fluoride during the first few years after eruption will encourage full maturation of the enamel. To counteract plaque stagnation and provide fluoride ions, it is crucially important to teach parents to brush erupting surfaces of first molars with special attention using fluoride toothpaste.

Another exception to the usually slow pace of lesion development occurs in high-risk patients (eg, those with compromised salivary flow). Patients who suffer from hyposalivation or a reduced quality of saliva are missing the protective clearance and buffering effects of saliva (see the article by Hara and Zero elsewhere in this issue for further exploration of this topic). This may lead to rapid and rampant lesion development. The calcium and phosphates from the saliva are the primary source for the recrystallizing minerals and thus for remineralization. Therefore, also in healthy individuals, stimulation of salivary flow by daily use of sugar-free chewing gum assists in caries management.

Changes in tooth structure

Teeth are composed of calcium phosphate minerals (hydroxyapatite) that dissolve when the pH drops below the critical value. The drop in pH necessary for demineralization in cementum and dentin (pH 6.2 to 6.7) is less than that required for enamel (pH 5.4 to 5.5).[12,13] Therefore, given the proper environment, both the initiation and progression of root surface caries lesions will occur more rapidly than in an enamel surface.[14] As the environmental pH recovers, the minerals precipitate on the remaining mineral crystals. Remineralization is slower than the dissolution process, but is still able to eliminate the damage done to tooth tissues by demineralization. If no or limited remineralization takes place, however, the demineralization will proceed, and a caries lesion will develop.

The dental caries process starts in the outer enamel and, as it proceeds, also involves and demineralizes dentin to a significant depth, even when the outer layer is still noncavitated. Low levels of fluoride are adequate for enamel remineralization but insufficient to facilitate dentin remineralization. The effect of the caries process in dentin is similar to that in enamel, except that dentin demineralizes at a higher pH and proceeds about twice as fast, because dentin has only half the mineral content of enamel. Even very deep lesions, extending through enamel into dentin, can be remineralized.[15] Although this is a slow process, it enlarges the window for noninvasive management and postponement of operative intervention for lesions that have passed the enamel–dentino junction.

Both initiation and progression of root surface caries lesions occur more rapidly in dentin than in coronal enamel.[4] Surface irregularities, collagen degradation, longer periods of acid challenge, and lower saliva clearance all aggravate the process of root caries. Taking the multitude of changes associated with aging into account, and the fact that root dentin is more prone to acid dissolution, it will be obvious that this will lead to differences in management strategy. Combating root caries may need greater fervor.

LESION ARREST AND REPAIR

Treatment and management strategies should be based on interpretation of activity of the lesion and future caries risk of the patient. Caries is a disease, caused by a multifactorial process, and contemporary caries management takes this into account. Current management approaches call for control of disease activity and tissue repair by reversal of mineral loss. Restorative treatment options are advised only when the caries disease process has resulted in more extensive damage (ie, cavitations), and form, function or esthetics need to be restored. The only (complementary) role restorations play in a patient's caries management plan is that they partially assist disease management by eliminating plaque stagnation spots and facilitate plaque control in case of clinically detected, frank cavitations.

In the very early active caries lesion (the *initial demineralized lesion*), only the external enamel microsurface is dissolved by plaque acids. After plaque removal, the ultrathin superficially eroded area will wear and become polished, changing its appearance from rough and chalky-white into a hard, shiny surface. When the lesion has progressed a little further and resulted in a deeper surface and subsurface disso-lution, it is called an *active noncavitated caries lesion*. Intervention in the caries process will now, in addition to the previously described initial process, also result in a slow remineralization of the subsurface defect. Although such remineralized lesions show a decrease in size (depth and width), they may remain visible as shiny, white lesions. The caries process has ceased, but the lesion is not completely recov-ered and may remain forever visible as white or brown scar tissue. Although they have not been reversed completely, these areas are more resistant to a subsequent caries attack than sound enamel. This will be explained in more detail subsequently when the mechanism of topical fluorides are discussed.

Special care must be taken with interpretation of radiographic evidence of deminer-alized tissue. An arrested, nonactive lesion may still present itself as a demineralized, radiolucent area on a radiograph. Such an arrested lesion, however, does not need any management and should be considered a tissue scar. Greater awareness of this phenomenon will help to reduce the perceived need for operative intervention and avoid overtreatment.

Assisting natural processes

The question now becomes how one can help naturally occurring processes to arrest lesion activity, respond to mineral dissolution by remineralization effort, and thus potentially reverse early caries lesions. Lesion activity can be halted with several means by taking the infectious part out of the equation. Diet modification, general or targeted antibacterial strategies, plaque-removal and plaque-reducing strategies, stimulation of salivary flow, and sealing of lesions, all lead to reduction or elimination of acid attacks on the tooth surface. This changes the dynamics of the ion exchange between the hard tissues and the ambient plaque fluids. In the presence of normal saliva, a reduction in demineralization automatically will result in remineralization, halting the caries process (see the article by Hara and Zero elsewhere in this issue for further exploration of this topic). An arrested lesion does not require treatment.

Basic Preventive Steps for Moderate/High Risk Patients		Special Needs
Patient motivation	Emphasize behavioral change	R + H
Diet counseling	Reduction of fermentable carbohydrate intake and frequency	R + H
	Reduction of softdrink consumption and frequency	R + H
Tooth brushing	Twice daily with fluoride toothpaste (preferably 3x/day)	R + H
Flossing	Daily, few times a week	R + H
Sugar-free gum	Chew 2 pieces for ≥5 min, 3 ×/d (after each meal preferred)	R + H
Sealants	All at-risk surfaces (sound or noncavitated)	H

Abbreviations: H, hyposalivation; R, root caries.

Plaque Reduction/Removal

The average speed of lesion progression on different surfaces has been determined.[16] Caries proceeds slowly on smooth surfaces (proximal and buccal/labial/lingual). Therefore, restorative intervention always should be postponed, and active preventive management and monitoring are indicated. This includes modifying the caries envi-ronment by improvement of oral hygiene (ie, twice-daily effective plaque removal and use of floss, diet modification, and provision of fluoride) (see the article by Hara and Zero elsewhere in this issue for further exploration of this topic). Although no good evidence exists for caries-preventive effect of tooth brushing alone, the conventional health wisdom keep your mouth clean is not only a social and cosmetic strategy. This tooth-cleaning advice will continue to be an important step in caries management for the foreseeable future, in particular when using fluoride toothpaste.

When lesions show cavitation, the caries process has not only reached the enamel–dentino junction, but the dentin is always involved.[17] Such lesions contain many cariogenic microorganisms and thus are by definition active lesions.[18] It is difficult to effectively remove plaque from these lesions, because access to the cavitation is problematic. Simply removing undermined and overhanging enamel margins from cavitated lesions will assist in keeping the lesion free from plaque. Open, accessible cavities, cleaned twice daily with fluoridated toothpaste, can be arrested and converted into a leathery or even hard lesion and lead to decreased activity and an arrested caries process.[19] This type of basic caries management, successful in the primary dentition, might be applicable to the permanent dentition as well when rampant caries require immediate and simple, noninvasive management. Carious dentitions can be managed so that the caries process is arrested, and the balance between physiologic de/remineralization processes has been reinstated.

Because cariogenic microflora thrive in bacterial plaque communities (ie, biofilm), reducing or disturbing their living environment is a sensible approach. Basic tooth cleaning is helpful in keeping the biomass of acidogenic and acid-tolerant microflora under control. Limiting available substrate for cariogenic bacteria by use of xylitol, for example, is another approach. Xylitol chewing gum is considered an adjunct preventive therapy that results in transient effect on the biofilm. The lack of well-designed randomized control trials (RCTs) results in a lack of definitive evidence for a caries-preventive effect of xylitol.[20]

The use of antibacterials like chlorhexidine (CHX) for caries prevention has been a controversial topic. The caries-inhibiting effect was not greater than fluoride, while CHX administration has several drawbacks (see the article by Svante Twetman elsewhere in this issue for further exploration of this topic). There is lack of consensus on evidence-based treatment protocols, and the evidence using different CHX modes and concentrations or a combined CHX-fluoride therapy is "suggestive but incomplete."[21] A recent meta-analysis on CHX-varnishes for targeted patient groups stated that there was either a nonsignificant effect or the effect was only shown in few studies.[22] Based on current inconclusive evidence, CHX rinse (0.12%) or varnish (1% CHX), the only products available in the United States, are not recommended for caries prevention. Even so, in spite of lacking wide consensus regarding efficacy, CHX use for short periods aiming to temporarily eliminate or reduce bacterial plaque may provide a complementary strategy in noninvasive management for high-caries risk individuals.

Nowadays, antibacterial strategies are no longer only wide spectrum therapies (eg, CHX) reducing biofilm and plaque formation. Promising, emerging research findings show positive effects of herbal and novel approaches targeting or modifying only the major cariogenic species in the biofilm communities. Probiotic approaches that retain the healthy benign plaque may define future strategies (see the article by Svante Twetman elsewhere in this issue for further exploration of this topic).

Brushing with fluoride toothpaste

Brushing teeth is still an excellent way to combine mechanical plaque removal with a therapeutic treatment. Brushing the plaque exposes the tooth surface to an environment that might mediate the initial caries process. Exposure of the surface to mineral-rich saliva may prevent mineral loss and induce mineral uptake if there are caries lesions in development. The use of fluoride toothpaste enhances the plaque removal effect by introducing fluoride ions at the clean surface during lesion development phase.

The effectiveness of fluoride increases when elevated levels are maintained throughout the day by frequent applications of small amounts of fluoride. The current understanding from numerous clinical trials, although of great complexity due to the number of variables, resulted in the widely accepted recommendation that *brushing at least twice daily with fluoride toothpaste* is appropriate for all age and risk groups. It is recommended to brush just before going to bed (to reduce plaque, remove remaining fermentable carbohydrates, and boost fluoride levels) and at one other time during the day at a mealtime. The recommendation for young children is supervised brushing and the use of a pea-size amount of fluoridated toothpaste (only when they can spit). Supervised brushing with 1000 ppm fluoride toothpaste resulted in 56% fewer decayed and filled surfaces in children compared with unsupervised children.[23]

Tooth Brushing	Special Needs
Tooth brushing (adults)	
Use over-the-counter fluoride toothpaste (approximately 1100 ppm fluoride)	
Brush at least twice a day (preferably 3×/d), including immediately before going to bed	
"Spit—don't rinse" should be the motto	
Tooth brushing in children:	
Supervise and check amount of toothpaste (pea-size) on brush, if at risk for fluorosis	
Finish-off brushing with special attention for occlusal surfaces of erupting teeth	Erupting surfaces

Special attention is needed when patients have appliances, and plaque removal becomes more difficult. Fixed and removable orthodontic appliances and partial dentures will encourage plaque retention and require special attention and motivation for plaque removal. The unbelievably high incidence of 73% of new white spot lesions during fixed orthodontic treatment presents a dire iatrogenic shortcoming in the profession.[24] In addition to motivational oral hygiene instruction and supplementary fluoride administration, monitoring compliance of these high caries risk patients (and intervene, when necessary) is a 'must' and a professional ethical responsibility.

Modifying ambient plaque/oral fluids

Increasing the amount of bioavailable ions in the saliva also will drive the remineralization process. Several caries management strategies rely on providing additional fluoride, calcium, or phosphate ions to saliva, with the intent to deliver an ample supply of ions to the immediate caries-active environment: the plaque–tooth interface.

Fluorides

Enamel crystals, the building blocks for enamel, consist of hydroxyapatite (HA). Therapeutic use of fluoride is aimed at substituting the HA crystals in the enamel with fluoroapatite (FA) and inhibition of the carbohydrate metabolism in the biofilm. When fluorides are present, the enamel crystals in the incipient lesion will be repaired or replaced with FA or fluorohydroxyapatite. These crystals are relatively insoluble.

Therefore repeated cycles of de/remineralization in the presence of fluorides result in a more caries-resistant enamel.[25] Presence of fluorides in the ambient solution effectively protects enamel during acid challenges. Therefore a frequent availability of fluoride ions in the oral fluids is important. In the early stages of a caries lesion, the bacterial acids in the surface biofilm penetrate through the eroded crystal spaces and form a porous mineral structure: the subsurface lesion. The mechanism by which fluoride inhibits demineralization is facilitating re-precipitation of dissolved calcium and phosphate ions on the remaining crystals. This mechanism prevents the tissue ions from being leached out to the environment into the plaque and saliva. Precipitated ions at the tooth surface decrease the pores in the enamel, obstruct the diffusion pathways for plaque acids, and hamper acid penetration into the enamel. When ambient pH is higher than approximately 5.5, fluoride will facilitate remineralization, promoting lesion arrest and enhancing repair.[26] On the other hand, a lack of fluoride constitutes a caries risk. The loss and incorporation of minerals in enamel is a continual dynamic process that takes place with and without fluoride. Frequent presence of fluorides at the tooth surface enhances this dynamic toward effective remineralization. To ensure high frequency of ion availability, the fluorides need to be replenished.

Retention of fluoride in the mouth is site-specific, and there is minimal transport of fluoride ions between left and right sides of the mouth or between arches. This explains also why localized lesions can occur while patients use fluoride toothpaste. A strong, off-label advice is thus to discourage vigorous rinsing with water after tooth brushing. Instead: encourage patients to only spit out the excess toothpaste, so that what remains will continue to facilitate remineralization processes. This no-rinse method resulted in 26% reduction in approximal caries incidence.[27]

Topical home fluorides: tooth pastes, mouth rinses, and gels

The use of fluoride toothpaste that retains a sufficient concentration of bioavailable fluoride is a cost-effective means of caries control. A recent summary of Cochrane systematic reviews on fluoride[28] concluded that the benefits of daily tooth brushing with fluoride toothpastes for preventing dental caries were firmly established, based on a sizeable body of evidence from randomized controlled trials. Although long-term studies in adults were still lacking,[29] a clear and similar effectiveness of topical fluoride toothpastes, mouth rinses, gels, and varnishes for preventing caries was confirmed.[30] The size of the reductions in caries increment in both the permanent and primary dentitions emphasizes the importance of including topical fluoride delivered through toothpastes, rinses, gels, or varnishes in any caries preventive program.[28]

After assessing the individual caries risk and fluoride exposure of a patient, the appropriate fluoride concentration should be considered. As a basic caries-preventive method, the concentration in over-the-counter (OTC) fluoride toothpastes in the United States is approximately 1100 ppm fluoride (for 7 years and older). The caries-preventive effect of regular use is typically 20% to 40% over 2 to 3 years.[31] In caries-active patients, it is essential to increase fluoride therapy until the caries is under control. This can be achieved by more intensive (at least three times per day) use of OTC fluoride toothpaste, asking the patient to refrain from rinsing after brushing or adding fluoride mouth rinses. Another therapeutic use of toothpaste is to apply the paste locally (with finger or brush) directly onto the cleaned active caries lesion before going to bed (taking advantage of the decreased salivary secretion at night). Alternatively, a prescription high-fluoride containing toothpaste (5000 ppm fluoride), fluoride rinses, or various professionally applied applications may be chosen. Compared with a conventional OTC toothpaste of 1100 ppm fluoride, a study in elders using 5000 ppm fluoride showed almost twice as much rehardening of noncavitated root lesions.[32]

A summary of seven systematic reviews concluded that additional caries reduction can be expected when another topical fluoride as mouth rinses, gels, and varnishes is combined with fluoride toothpaste.[29] Home fluoride rinses may benefit adults with active caries who have difficulty cleaning their teeth adequately. Rinses with 0.02% NaF (US market) should be used daily for a full minute. Prescription solutions with 0.2% NaF may be used daily or weekly, depending on the caries risk of the patient. Products without alcohol are preferred to avoid dry-mouth effects.

Adjunct Topical Therapies for Moderate/High Risk Patients	Special Needs
Home fluoride options:	
Prescription fluoride toothpaste: 5000 ppm F	R + H
Brush at least twice a day (preferably 3x/day), incl. immediately before going to bed	
"Spit—don't rinse" should be the motto	
Daily (in tray – radiation hyposalivation)	H
Fluoride rinses	
Twice daily/daily/weekly (depending on need and product)	R + H
In-office fluoride options:	
Fluoride gels/foams: 1.23% APF or neutral 2% NaF	
4 min, 2–4× per year	
4× over 2–4 weeks (root caries)	R + H
Fluoride varnishes:	
Isolate each quadrant with cotton rolls	
Apply to lesions and other surfaces at risk	
2–4× per year depending on subject's risk	R + H

Abbreviations: H, hyposalivation; R, root caries.

Professionally applied/in-office topical fluoride applications

To further assist the body's response to caries attacks and address mineral imbalances, several professionally applied preventive measures are available, such as topical application of concentrated fluoride solutions, gels, or varnishes. To achieve optimal caries-preventive effect, the more frequent elevated fluoride levels are offered, the better. Thus, the intensity of home-used fluoride may have to be stepped up for a while by adding a third fluoride boost per day through extra brushing with high-concentration fluoride toothpaste, a fluoride rinse, or other forms (ie, tablets, gels).

Professional application of topical fluorides is an effective approach to caries control, as supported by strong evidence from many clinical trials. The American Dental Association (ADA) Council on Scientific Affairs developed evidence-based clinical recommendations for professionally applied topical fluoride, summarized in this paragraph and in the **Table 1**.[33] Strong evidence (grade A) supports its use for moderate and high caries risk children and adolescents (younger than 18 years). Although there are no clinical trials with adults, there is reason to believe that fluoride gels and varnishes work similarly for adults in these risk categories (grade D). As can be seen in the table, low-risk individuals may not receive additional benefits from professionally applied topical fluoride application (grade B). Fluoride gels and foam should be applied for 4 minutes. A 1-minute fluoride application was not endorsed, as clinical equivalence was not proven. The Council on Scientific Affairs found insufficient evidence to address whether there is a difference in efficacy between sodium fluoride (NaF) and acidulated phosphate fluoride (APF) gels.

Based on systematic reviews, an evidence-based protocol for the use of fluoride varnish in children and adolescents recommends that fluoride varnishes (in the United States 5% NaF) should be applied twice a year, unless the individual has no risk of caries.[34] There is also good evidence of the complementary efficacy of preventive strategies such as sealants and varnish, as well as tooth brushing.[34] Fluoride toothpastes in comparison to mouth rinses or gels appear to have a similar degree of effectiveness for the prevention of dental caries in children. Fluoride varnish was not more effective than mouth rinses, and the evidence for the comparative effectiveness of fluoride varnishes and gels, and mouth rinses and gels is inconclusive.[29]

Caries-active patients In addition to a fluoride regimen at home, the caries-active patient may benefit from topical fluoride applications, which may be repeated every 2 to 3 months until caries activity is under control. In-office applications, however, are time-consuming and thus not as cost-effective, unless used in high caries-active patients.

Erupting teeth *Mineralization of erupting teeth*, following exposure of immature enamel to saliva, is a natural physiologic process.[35] Maturation can be stimulated by providing an oral environment that is supersaturated with ions. Hence, at times of tooth eruption (5 to 6 years of age; and 12 to 13 years of age) special attention is warranted for cleaning erupting surfaces and providing additional topical fluorides.[36] In addition to application of topical fluorides, erupting surfaces also may be protected by a transitional glass ionomer sealant. In contrast with resin sealants, glass ionomer may be used when moisture control is a problem. Recent meta-analysis found no conclusive evidence that either glass ionomer or resin-based sealant was superior to the other in preventing dental caries.[37] Glass ionomer sealant is indicated for erupting occlusal surfaces with overlying operculum where continued mineralization is needed. Upon setting, glass ionomer introduces an acidic cariostatic environment and provides a fluoride boost to the underlying maturing enamel. Serving as a semipermeable membrane, and replenished by fluoride toothpaste, it may continue to provide fluoride ions to the enamel during the eruption period while concurrently protecting the surface from acidic plaque fluids.

Root caries *Active root caries lesions* can be arrested by effective daily plaque removal with fluoride toothpaste.[38,39] The quality of plaque removal, and thus exposure of incipient lesions to saliva, is crucial for arresting active caries root lesions; buccal and lingual surfaces showed about 50% success rate, with less favorable outcome for approximal root lesions.[38] Application of topical fluoride, independent of the mode chosen, is appropriate management for root lesions.[40] This can be complemented with a 2-week regimen of twice-daily 0.12% chlorhexidine rinse, or in-office CHX varnish (currently in the United States only available as 1% CHX/1% thymol varnish). Patients also may be advised to use daily xylitol chewing gum (see the article by Svante Twetman elsewhere in this issue for further exploration of this topic).

Hyposalivation *Patients with a dry mouth*, or those who have been exposed to radiotherapy of salivary glands inevitably develop rampant, raging caries, unless following a strict caries-control program. As soon as radiotherapy begins, daily self-applied 5 minute topical applications with a 1% NaF gel in individually fitted trays[41] are advised in addition to meticulous daily plaque removal (brushing, flossing). Disclosing

Table 1
In-office topical fluorides

Evidence-Based Clinical Recommendations for Professionally Applied Topical Fluoride

Risk Category	Age Category for Recall Patients					
	<6 years		6 to 18 years		18 + years	
	Recommendation	Strength[a]	Recommendation	Strength[a]	Recommendation	Strength[a]
Low	May not receive additional benefit from professional topical fluoride application[b]	B	May not receive additional benefit from professional topical fluoride application[b]	B	May not receive additional benefit from professional topical fluoride application[b]	D
Moderate	Varnish application at 6-month intervals	A	Varnish application at 6-month intervals or Fluoride gel application at 6-month intervals	A	Varnish application at 6-month intervals or Fluoride gel application at 6-month intervals	D[e] D[d]

	Recommendation	Strength	Recommendation	Strength	Recommendation	Strength
High	Varnish application at 6-month intervals	A	Varnish application at 6-month intervals	A	Varnish application at 6-month intervals	D[e]
	or		or		or	
	Varnish application at 3-month intervals	D[c]	Varnish application at 3-month intervals	A[c]	Varnish application at 3-month intervals	D[e]
			or		or	
			Fluoride gel application at 6-month intervals	A	Fluoride gel application at 6-month intervals	D[d]
			or		or	
			Fluoride gel application at 3-month intervals	D[d]	Fluoride gel application at 3-month intervals	D[d]

Laboratory data demonstrate foam's equivalence to gels in terms of fluoride release; however, only two clinical trials have been published evaluating its effectiveness. Because of this, the recommendations for use of fluoride varnish and gel have not been extrapolated to foams.

Because there is insufficient evidence to address whether there is a difference in the efficacy of sodium fluoride versus acidulated phosphate fluoride gels, the clinical recommendations do not specify between these two formulations of fluoride gels. Application time for fluoride gel and foam should be 4 minutes. A 1-minute fluoride application is not endorsed.

[a] Strength of recommendation ranges from A (highest level of evidence from systematic reviews of randomized controlled trials) to D (lowest level of evidence from expert committee reports or opinions or clinical experience of respected authorities).

[b] Fluoridated water and fluoride toothpastes may provide adequate caries prevention in this risk category. Whether to apply topical fluoride in such cases is a decision that should balance this consideration with the practitioner's professional judgment and the individual patient's preferences.

[c] Emerging evidence indicates that applications more frequent than twice per year may be more effective in preventing caries.

[d] Although there are no clinical trials, there is reason to believe that fluoride gels would work similarly in this age group.

[e] Although there are no clinical trials, there is reason to believe that fluoride varnish would work similarly in this age group.

remaining plaque, every day after brushing, to complete its removal may assist in achieving this meticulous daily plaque control that is so crucial for a positive outcome. If plaque control is insufficient, twice-daily fluoride (0.05% NaF) rinses could be added. Alternatively, in an attempt to temporarily boost plaque control, a dual rinsing strategy of fluoride and CHX-gluconate (0.05% NaF with 0.2% CHX) rinse could be advised to concurrently suppress the oral microflora. However, it is recommended to separate the application of an anionic product such as fluoride and a cationic product like CHX by at least a few hours to avoid binding of the active ingredients, and they should never be mixed together for the same reason. It is wise to provide regular professional tooth cleaning to these patients followed by high-concentration in-office topical fluoride application. Calcium phosphate-based compounds also may have a beneficial effect for patients with hyposalivation.[42,43]

Potentially Helpful Adjuncts to Home Fluoride (Emerging)	Special Needs
Antimicrobial boost: 4–6 ×/year	
Xylitol chewing gum: xylitol as first ingredient	
Chew 2 pieces for ≥5 min, 3×/day (after each meal preferred) for 2 weeks	
CHX rinse: 0.12% CHX-gluconate	Hyposalivation
Rinse ½ oz for 30 s, 2×/day for 2 weeks	
Calcium-based therapy:	
Calcium-based products (eg, paste, toothpaste, mints) with/without fluoride	Hyposalivation
Depending on product	

Calcium-Based Strategies

Fluoride alone cannot achieve remineralization; calcium and phosphate ions are necessary for remineralization to occur. The calcium and phosphates in saliva are the primary source for recrystallizing minerals. When salivary flow is hampered, rampant caries is the effect of the lack of these minerals. Remineralizing agents seek to promote remineralization through increase of bioavailable calcium and phosphate ions that become incorporated in tooth structure. Supplementing calcium and phosphates is likely to have a positive effect, in particular when effective fluoride levels are available at the same time. Although various formulations and modes have been tested in vitro, the complexity of the oral environment with/without saliva might lead to different results. With normal salivary flow, sufficient amounts of mineral will be readily available, and additional minerals may not be helpful. On the contrary, too much calcium, phosphate, or fluoride may contribute to limited remineralization.[44] With hyposalivation, however, supplementing fluorides with home applications of amorphous and reactive calcium phosphate complexes may greatly assist remineralization.

Potential benefits have been shown for casein phosphopeptides, amorphous calcium phosphates, and other approaches. Inhibition of enamel and dentin demineralization, promotion of remineralization, and a slow-down of the caries process as well as regression of subsurface lesions have been reported for casein phosphopeptide–amorphous calcium phosphate (CCP-ACP).[45] Although a remineralizing effect is reported for chewing gum and mints with CPP-ACP, solid evidence to support clinical efficacy for specific delivery modes remains lacking. More well-designed and independent studies investigating clinically relevant conditions are needed. A recent systematic review reported that the quantity and quality of clinical trial evidence were insufficient to make conclusions regarding the long-term effectiveness of casein derivatives, specifically CPP-ACP, in preventing caries in vivo.[46] Clinical studies investigating the clinical benefits of CCP-ACP paste with and without fluoride are promising and emerging.[47] Although persuasive scientific evidence from randomized clinical trials (RCTs) is not yet available,[48] the off-label use of CPP-ACP technology may hold potential as an adjunct to fluoride treatment in the noninvasive management of early caries lesions.

Calcium sodium phosphosilicate bioactive glass is another new agent that reacts with an aqueous environment and releases calcium and phosphate ions. It is used as a desensitizer and approved as hypersensitivity agent. Off-label use as remineralizing agent is promoted, but simultaneous delivery of the right amounts of calcium, phosphate, and fluoride ions at the same time and location might be problematic and cause undesired adverse effects (eg, rapid precipitation). More research is needed to provide scientific evidence supporting claims of caries prevention and remineralization.[44]

Other emerging calcium-based strategies are entering the market. These include calcium phosphate solutions to reduce root caries and ACP technologies that can remineralize hard tooth tissues or at a minimum slow down the demineralization process.[49] Second-generation ACPs and multimodal approaches are being developed to prevent caries. These include new compounds with antimicrobial and remineralization potential.[50] In addition, a new experimental product employing synthetic HA in an acid paste is said to repair defects and replace crystals within a matter of minutes.[51] These strategies, however, are only recently available, too recent to be supported by solid evidence of their anticaries efficacy.

Summarizing, at this moment the scientific evidence to support the claim of caries-preventive efficacy from calcium-based products available in the US market has not been provided. Although promising in some cases and potentially beneficial, few studies have confirmed calcium-based agents have actually resulted in an anticaries benefit. Combinations of fluoride and calcium-based ingredients may involve potential formulation and compatibility challenges, and their mechanisms of action are likely difficult to demonstrate.[52] The level of evidence for calcium-based strategies reported in the literature remains incomplete and insufficient to substantiate claims by manufacturers or researchers. Application of these products cannot yet be recommended as evidence-based caries-preventive measures.

THE PROVEN AND THE NEW
Resin Sealants—A Proven Effective Management Strategy

An increasing body of evidence indicates that arrest of lesions is possible, even when dentin is involved. Sealants protect the underlying surface by blocking renewed and continuous attacks by plaque acids. Sealants prevent plaque accumulation and dissolution of minerals from the tooth tissues. They have been used successfully for many years[53,54] and have shown a clear benefit even when partially lost.[55,56] In particular when caries risk is moderate to high, teeth with caries-susceptible pits and fissures will greatly benefit from sealing. The ADA Council on Scientific Affairs assessed the available body of evidence, which led to clinical recommendations.[57] The effectiveness of sealants in managing noncavitated and cavitated caries lesions was overwhelming.[58] The recommendations were based on six systematic reviews, and no matter how studies were grouped, the effect of sealants was strong and consistent. Sealed noncavitated lesions consistently had better outcomes than unsealed lesions, while the percentage of sealed carious surfaces that progressed was low. Sealants resulted in a caries reduction of about 71% up to 5 years after placement.[58]

Concerns about placing sealants over undetected dentin caries are ungrounded, as there is ample evidence that caries lesions do not progress as long as the fissures remain sealed.[59,60] It also has been reported that sealed teeth with fissures showing a partial sealant or a lost sealant over a 3-year period still showed caries reduction, and thus were more protected than unsealed teeth.[61] The caries risk in formerly sealed teeth appeared to be not higher than teeth that never were sealed.[56] Sealing of cavitated lesions significantly reduced bacteria levels (50% to 99% of mean bacteria counts), and this effect increased with time.[62] Caries lesions under intact sealants may even regress. Cavitated, but sealed frank dentin caries lesions also have been shown not to progress over a period of 10 years.[63] Additionally, sealed restorations placed over caries lesions arrested the caries progression in these lesions.[64] Recently, updated evidence-based recommendations were published by a Centers for Disease Control and Prevention (CDC) work group, recommending to seal sound surfaces and noncavitated lesions and to provide sealants to children even if follow-up cannot be ensured.[65]

Because even active dentin lesions that are covered by a well-applied sealant do not progress, there is no good reason to be hesitant in promoting sealants in caries-prone patients. Sealant protection is in particular indicated during periods of tooth eruption (ages 5 to 6 years and 10 to 12 years). When moisture control is a problem, glass ionomer sealants may be indicated for erupting first molars. Also older high-risk patients with suspect fissures will benefit from sealants. A third category of high-risk patients, those with appliances, also will benefit greatly from sealing tooth areas with a high potential of future caries activity (eg, around orthodontic brackets and removable partial denture clasps).

As strongly evidenced, both sealing of the caries process and sealing of restorations appear to be highly effective in conserving sound tooth tissue and providing protection to the hard tooth tissues against caries progression. Where indicated (patients with moderate and high caries risk), sealant application is an essential part of an effective and preventive caries management plan. Only when previous attempts to arrest the lesion have failed and there is evidence of lesion progression is a restorative treatment approach warranted.

Resin infiltration of lesions

Resin infiltration of early lesions is a recent development by which subsurface porosities in the lesion are being filled with a resin to strengthen this area.[66] Due to the concurrent sealing of the caries lesion from the oral environment, progression of the lesion is halted. Once the porous demineralized enamel is filled with resin, it has been claimed that its refractory index changes also. The lesion may become less opaque and thus less visible as it regains translucency. After erosion of the superficial surface layer using hydrochloric acid, the underlying pores are opened up, and a low-viscosity resin is able to penetrate into the demineralized tissues. A drawback of this technique is the need for erosion of the intact surface layer, which ultimately is replaced by the resin and the fact that the resin, once placed, will make natural remineralization therapy impossible (similar to a sealant). Short-term results from the first clinical studies that used this enticing concept for approximal and smooth surface lesions are emerging, and judgment about its clinical efficacy is still out. Until proper clinical trials have been presented, this novel approach should be used wisely and in conjunction with other preventive strategies.

Alternative Treatment Options

In the last decade, laser ablation has been applied in caries research. Lasers have been used to coalesce enamel fissures[67] and to provide greater caries resistance to the outer enamel surface. Increased attention for this technology has led to research aiming to optimize the laser parameters to achieve an optimal ablation effect. The large variability in lasers and laser parameters used has not yet led to consensus about their use.[67,68] CO_2 laser irradiation in combination with fluoride treatment is more effective in inhibiting caries-like lesions than CO_2 laser irradiation or fluoride alone.[69] These technologies are still emerging, and evidence of clinical anticariogenic efficacy is not yet available or scarce at best. No evidence of anticaries efficacy in controlled clinical studies has been reported so far. Laser treatments for caries inhibition are still considered experimental and cannot be recommended.

An interesting discussion of other novel preventive management options that are currently under investigation includes promising treatments already applied in clinical practice.[70] The authors conclude that many of the techniques mentioned show considerable promise, and dentists should be aware of these developments and follow their progress. The evidence, however, for each of these novel preventive treatment options is currently insufficient to make widespread recommendations, and more research needs to be done to show clinical efficacy for effective caries control.

SUMMARY

At the individual patient level, there is a great variation in the complex interplay between all known and unknown factors that are involved in lesion development. Assessment of caries risk of the individual patient is an important prerequisite for an appropriate and successful management strategy. Therefore, clinical recommendations have to be balanced with the clinician's professional judgement and the patient's history and preference.

Available strategies for noninvasive tissue repair are summarized in **Table 2**. By providing repair options that encourage remineralization, the damage of the initial caries process may be healed. Vulnerable tissues may be protected and strengthened.

Noninvasive Management Strategies—Implications for Clinical Care

Evidence-based management strategy should be tailored to the individual, with due regard to negative risk factors.

Find out which major causal factors led to the patient's caries problem. To prioritize and address these factors should be the main goals when assisting the body's response toward caries control.

Table 2
Protection and remineralization of damaged enamel

Noninvasive Demineralized Tissue Repair		
Mode	**Mechanism**	**Strategy**
Remineralize	Replenish ions (F, Ca, P)	Heal + increase acid resistance
Remineralize + protect	Seal lesion area (glass ionomer)	Heal + seal
Protect	Seal lesion area (resin)	Seal
Strengthen + protect	Resin infiltrant	Strengthen + seal

Sealants are strongly recommended for all at-risk surfaces (sound or noncavitated)

Management strategies should be based on interpretation of lesion activity and future caries risk of the patient.

Active monitoring of lesion activity and the patient's compliance with behavioral modifications (oral hygiene, adjunct therapies, and diet) are essential parts of a successful caries management and maintenance plan.

Preventive noninvasive strategies demand and rely on patient cooperation. Regular recall visits to assess and discuss cooperation are important for long-term results. Motivating the patient is key to success!

Although there are increasing numbers of technologies aimed at enhancing tooth remineralization, fluoride remains the most widely used agent for managing the caries process, supported by strong levels of evidence.

The primary modes of action of fluorides are enhancing remineralization, inhibiting demineralization, and inhibition of the biofilm. The most important effect, enhancement of remineralization, only can occur in the presence of calcium and phosphate ions.

When saliva flow is inadequate, topical fluorides might be assisted by additional supply of calcium and phosphates to enhance remineralization.

In individuals with a high caries challenge, fluoride therapy is not always enough to overcome the challenge. In high-risk individuals, an effective management strategy may call for increased and frequent fluoride delivery together with an antimicrobial therapy to take advantage of the synergy and complementary effect of both modes of action.

New emerging technologies should be considered adjuncts to fluoride treatments until their caries-preventive and therapeutic efficacy is sufficiently evidenced in well-designed RCTs.

REFERENCES

1. Peters MC, McLean ME. Minimally invasive operative care. Part 1: minimum intervention and concepts for minimally invasive cavities. J Adhes Dent 2001;3:7–16.
2. Lagerløf F, Oliveby A. Clinical implications: new strategies for caries treatment. In: Stookey G, editor. Early detection of dental caries. Indianapolis: Indiana University School of Dentistry; 1996. p. 297–321.
3. Shwartz M, Gröndhal HG, Pliskin JS, et al. A longitudinal analysis from bitewing radiographs of the rate of progression of proximal carious lesions through human dental enamel. Arch Oral Biol 1984;29:529–36.
4. Gröndhal HG, Hollender L, Malmcrona E, et al. Dental caries and restorations in teenagers. II. A longitudinal radiographic study of the caries increment of proximal surfaces among urban teenagers in Sweden. Swed Dent J 1977;1:51–7.
5. Mejàre I, Källestal C, Stenlund H, et al. Caries development from 11 to 22 years of age: a prospective radiographic study. Prevalence and distribution. Caries Res 1998;32:10–6.
6. Hyatt TP. Observable and unobservable pits and fissures. Dent Cosmos 1931;73: 586–92.
7. Creanor SL, Russell JI, Strang DM, et al. The prevalence of clinically undetected occlusal dentine caries in Scottish adolescents. Br Dent J 1990;169:126–9.
8. Weerheijm KL, Kidd EA, Groen HJ. The effect of fluoridation on the occurrence of hidden caries in clinically sound occlusal surfaces. Caries Res 1997;31: 30–4.

9. Machiulskiene V, Nyvad B, Baelum V. A comparison of clinical and radiographic caries diagnoses in posterior teeth of 12-year-old Lithuanian children. Caries Res 1999;33(5):340–8.
10. Seow WK. Pre-eruptive intracoronal resorption as an entity of occult caries. Pediatr Dent 2000;22:370–6.
11. Stenlund H, Mejàre I, Källestål C. Caries rates related to approximal caries at ages 11–13: a 10-year follow-up study in Sweden. J Dent Res 2002;81(7): 455–8.
12. Hoppenbrouwers PM, Driessens FC, Borggreven JM. The mineral solubility of human tooth roots. Arch Oral Biol 1987;32(5):319–22.
13. Atkinson JC, Wu AJ. Salivary gland dysfunction: causes, symptoms, treatment. J Am Dent Assoc 1994;125(4):409–16.
14. Dung TZ, Liu AH. Molecular pathogenesis of root dentin caries. Oral Dis 1999; 5(2):92–9.
15. Ten Cate JM, Damen JJM, Buijs MJ. Inhibition of dentin remineralisation by fluoride in vitro. Caries Res 1998;32:141–7.
16. Pitts NB, Kidd EAM. The prescription and timing of bite wing radiography in the management of dental caries. Br Dent J 1992;172:225–7.
17. Ekstrand KR, Kuzmina I, Bjørndal L, et al. Relationship between external and histologic features of progressive stages of caries in the occlusal fossa. Caries Res 1995;29(4):243–50.
18. Angmar-Mànsson B, Al-Khateeb S, Tranaeus S. Monitoring the caries process. Optical methods for clinical diagnosis and quantification of enamel caries. Eur J Oral Sci 1996;104(4):480–5.
19. Nyvad B, Fejerskov O. Active root surface caries converted into inactive caries as a response to oral hygiene. Scand J Dent Res 1986;94(3):281–4.
20. Twetman S. Current controversies—is there merit? Adv Dent Res 2009;21(1): 48–52.
21. Autio-Gold J. The role of chlorhexidine in caries prevention. Oper Dent 2008; 33(6):710–6.
22. Twetman S, Stecksén-Blicks C. Probiotics and oral health effects in children. Int J Paediatr Dent 2008;18(1):3–10.
23. Curnow MM, Pine CM, Burnside G, et al. A randomised controlled trial of the efficacy of supervised toothbrushing in high-caries-risk children. Caries Res 2002; 36(4):294–300.
24. Richter AE, Arruda AO, Peters MC, et al. Incidence of caries lesions among patients treated with comprehensive orthodontics. Am J Orthod Dentofacial Orthop 2010;137, in press.
25. Featherstone JDB. Prevention and reversal of dental caries: role of low-level fluoride. Community Dent Oral Epidemiol 1999;27:31–40.
26. Hausen H. Benefits of topical fluorides firmly established. Evid Based Dent 2004; 5:36–7.
27. Sjögren K, Birkhed D, Rangmar B. Effect of a modified toothpaste technique on approximal caries in preschool children. Caries Res 1995;29(6):435–41.
28. Marinho VC. Cochrane reviews of randomized trials of fluoride therapies for preventing dental caries. Eur Arch Paediatr Dent 2009;10(3):183–91.
29. Twetman S, Axelsson S, Dahlgren H, et al. Caries-preventive effect of fluoride toothpaste: a systematic review. Acta Odontol Scand 2003;61(6): 347–55.
30. Marinho VC, Higgins JP, Sheiham A, et al. One topical fluoride (toothpastes, or mouthrinses, or gels, or varnishes) versus another for preventing dental

caries in children and adolescents. Cochrane Database Syst Rev 2004;(1): CD002780.

31. Clarkson JE, Ellwood RP, Chandler RE. A comprehensive summary of fluoride dentifrice caries clinical trials. Am J Dent 1993;6:S59–106.

32. Baysan A, Lynch E, Ellwood R, et al. Reversal of primary root caries using dentifrices containing 5000 and 1100 ppm fluoride. Caries Res 2001;35(1):41–6.

33. American Dental Association Council on Scientific Affairs. Professionally applied topical fluoride: evidence-based clinical recommendations. J Am Dent Assoc 2006;137(8):1151–9.

34. Azarpazhooh A, Main PA. Fluoride varnish in the prevention of dental caries in children and adolescents: a systematic review. J Can Dent Assoc 2008;74(1):73–9.

35. Crabb HS, Darling AI. The gradient of mineralization in developing enamel. Arch Oral Biol 1960;52:118–22.

36. Etty EJ, Henneberke M, Gruythuysen RJ, et al. Influence of oral hygiene on early enamel caries. Caries Res 1994;28(2):132–6.

37. Yengopal V, Mickenautsch S, Bezerra AC, et al. Caries-preventive effect of glass ionomer and resin-based fissure sealants on permanent teeth: a meta analysis. J Oral Sci 2009;51(3):373–82.

38. Emilson CG, Ravald N, Birkhed D. Effects of a 12-month prophylactic programme on selected oral bacterial populations on root surfaces with active and inactive carious lesions. Caries Res 1993;27(3):195–200.

39. Burgess JO, Gallo JR. Treating root-surface caries. Dent Clin North Am 2002; 46(2):385–404.

40. Heijnsbroek M, Paraskevas S, Van der Weijden GA. Fluoride interventions for root caries: a review. Oral Health Prev Dent 2007;5(2):145–52.

41. Dreizen S, Brown LR, Daly TE, et al. Prevention of xerostomia-related dental caries in irradiated cancer patients. J Dent Res 1977;56(2):99–104.

42. Llena C, Forner L, Baca P. Anticariogenicity of casein phosphopeptide-amorphous calcium phosphate: a review of the literature. J Contemp Dent Pract 2009;10(3):1–9.

43. Singh ML, Papas AS. Long-term clinical observation of dental caries in salivary hypofunction patients using a supersaturated calcium-phosphate remineralizing rinse. J Clin Dent 2009;20(3):87–92.

44. Wefel JS. NovaMin: likely clinical success. Adv Dent Res 2009;21(1):40–3.

45. Reynolds EC. Casein phosphopeptide-amorphous calcium phosphate: the scientific evidence. Adv Dent Res 2009;21(1):25–9.

46. Azarpazhooh A, Limeback H. Clinical efficacy of casein derivatives: a systematic review of the literature. J Am Dent Assoc 2008;139(7):915–24, [quiz 94–5].

47. Bailey DL, Adams GG, Tsao CE, et al. Regression of postorthodontic lesions by a remineralizing cream. J Dent Res 2009;88(12):1148–53.

48. Zero DT. Recaldent—evidence for clinical activity. Adv Dent Res 2009;21(1):30–4.

49. Chow LC, Vogel GL. Enhancing remineralization. Oper Dent 2001;26(Suppl 6): 27–38.

50. Tung MS, Eichmiller FC. Amorphous calcium phosphates for tooth mineralization. Compend Contin Educ Dent 2004;25:9–13.

51. Yamagishi K, Onuma K, Suzuki T, et al. Materials chemistry: a synthetic enamel for rapid tooth repair. Nature 2005;433(7028):819.

52. Pfarrer AM, Karlinsey RL. Challenges of implementing new remineralization technologies. Adv Dent Res 2009;21(1):79–82.

53. Simonsen RJ. Retention and effectiveness of dental sealant after 15 years. J Am Dent Assoc 1991;122:34–42.

54. Heller KE, Reed SG, Bruner FW, et al. Longitudinal evaluation of sealing molars with and without incipient dental caries in a public health program. J Public Health Dent 1995;55(3):148–53.
55. Messer LB, Calache H, Morgan MV. The retention of pit and fissure sealants placed in primary school children by Dental Health Services, Victoria. Aust Dent J 1997;42(4):233–9.
56. Griffin SO, Gray SK, Malvitz DM, et al. Caries risk in formerly sealed teeth. J Am Dent Assoc 2009;140(4):415–23.
57. Beauchamp J, Caufield PW, Crall JJ, et al. Evidence-based clinical recommendations for the use of pit-and-fissure sealants: a report of the American Dental Association Council on Scientific Affairs. J Am Dent Assoc 2008;139:257–68.
58. Griffin SO, Oong E, Kohn W, et al. The effectiveness of sealants in managing caries lesions. J Dent Res 2008;87(2):169–74.
59. Handelman S. The effect of sealant placement on occlusal caries progression. Clin Prev Dent 1982;4:11–6.
60. Mertz-Fairhurst EJ, Schuster GS, Fairhurst CW. Arresting caries by sealants: results of a clinical study. J Am Dent Assoc 1986;112:194–8.
61. Handelman SL, Leverett DH, Iker HP. Longitudinal radiographic evaluation of the progress of caries under sealants. J Pedod 1985;9:119–26.
62. Oong EM, Griffin SO, Kohn WG, et al. The effect of dental sealants on bacteria levels in caries lesions: a review of the evidence. J Am Dent Assoc 2008;139: 271–8.
63. Mertz-Fairhurst E, Curtis J, Ergle JW, et al. Ultraconservative and cariostatic sealed restorations: results at year 10. J Am Dent Assoc 1998;129:55–66.
64. Briley JB, Dove SB, Mertz-Fairhurst EJ, et al. Computer-assisted densitometric image analysis (CADIA) of previously sealed carious teeth: a pilot study. Oper Dent 1997;22:105–14.
65. Gooch BF, Griffin SO, Gray SK, et al. Preventing dental caries through school-based sealant programs: updated recommendations and reviews of evidence. J Am Dent Assoc 2009;140(11):1356–65.
66. Paris S, Meyer-Lueckel H. Inhibition of caries progression by resin infiltration in situ. Caries Res 2010;44(1):47–54.
67. Myaki SI, Watanabe IS, Eduardo CP, et al. Nd:YAG laser effects on the occlusal surface of premolars. Am J Dent 1998;11(3):103–5.
68. Esteves-Oliveira M, Zezell DM, Meister J, et al. CO_2 Laser (10.6 microm) parameters for caries prevention in dental enamel. Caries Res 2009;43(4):261–8.
69. Rodrigues LK, Nobre dos Santos M, Pereira D, et al. Carbon dioxide laser in dental caries prevention. J Dent Res 2004;32(7):531–40.
70. Longbottom C, Ekstrand K, Zero D, et al. Novel preventive treatment options. Monogr Oral Sci 2009;21:156–63.

Treatment Protocols: Nonfluoride Management of the Caries Disease Process and Available Diagnostics

Svante Twetman, DDS, Odont Dr[a,b,]*

KEYWORDS

- Caries • Chlorhexidine • Lactobacilli • Mutans streptococci
- Saliva • Xylitol • Probiotics

Dental caries forms through a complex interaction over time between acid-producing bacteria and fermentable carbohydrate, and many host factors including teeth and saliva.[1] The process can be described as a dynamic balance between re- and demineralization; if more minerals are lost than gained from the hard tissues over time, a lesion occurs as a sign of the disease.[2] The acids that dissolve the dental hard tissues are produced by bacteria that are general members of the commensal microflora. Therefore, an antibacterial approach to manage caries by controlling or removing bacteria is a key issue in the modern noninvasive medical model of caries treatment. But it is not only the amount of oral bacteria that counts. According to the ecological plaque hypothesis,[3] a caries-inductive environment gives rise to changes in the composition of the biofilm. During periods of constant pH stress, highly acid-producing and acid-tolerating species have an ecological advantage that results in a simplification of the biofilm diversity. Consequently, acid-tolerant microorganisms such as mutans streptococci, lactobacilli, and yeasts are considered as markers of a caries-promoting environment rather than direct and sole causative organisms. The key to modern caries management is to counteract rapid decreases in pH in the dental biofilm and maintain a neutral environment that promotes microbial homeostasis. This article reviews the evidence for some common antibacterial concepts with potential to benefit the biofilm

[a] Department of Cariology and Endodontics, Institute of Odontology, Faculty of Health Sciences, University of Copenhagen, Nørre Allé 20, DK-2200 Copenhagen N, Denmark
[b] Maxillofacial Unit, County Hospital, SE-30185 Halmstad, Sweden
* Department of Cariology and Endodontics, Institute of Odontology, Faculty of Health Sciences, University of Copenhagen, Nørre Allé 20, DK-2200 Copenhagen N, Denmark.
E-mail address: stwe@sund.ku.dk

Dent Clin N Am 54 (2010) 527–540
doi:10.1016/j.cden.2010.03.009
0011-8532/10/$ – see front matter © 2010 Elsevier Inc. All rights reserved.

EVIDENCE FOR SALIVARY DIAGNOSTICS IN CARIES ACTIVITY ASSESSMENT

Although it is obvious that saliva plays a significant role in the caries process, the benefits of salivary diagnostics for the individual patient are not clear-cut.[6] Threshold limits may vary among different individuals and the so-called normal values for flow rate are more reliable in populations than among individuals for screening purposes. In spite of extensive research on the topic in recent decades, systematic reviews are still rare. There is good evidence to suggest that presence of mutans streptococci in saliva of young caries-free children is associated with a considerable increased caries risk.[7] The findings concerning lactobacilli, however, are contradictory and less conclusive.[8] Among the nonmicrobial variables, salivary flow rate is the most important single parameter, whereas the buffer effect shows only a weak negative association with caries activity.[5] Furthermore, a significant association between one or more saliva factors and caries established in cross-sectional studies does not mean that those factors are useful as predictors.[6] The diagnostic or predictive value of saliva tests must be evaluated in prospective longitudinal studies, and further research is required to eradicate the questions concerning its clinical routine use.

ANTIMICROBIAL AND ANTISEPTIC APPROACHES

Although tooth cleaning is probably the most common way of eliminating bacteria, the focus in this article is on topical applications of chemotherapeutic agents and measures that may interfere with the caries balance. When evaluating the evidence for treatment effects, it is important to distinguish between results obtained with microbial or clinical end points. The former are called intermediate or surrogate end points because they may be indicative from an evidence-based point of view. For example, numerous good-quality trials convincingly show significant mutans streptococci suppression after chlorhexidine (CHX) therapy, but the studies reporting the effect on lesion incidence and control are fewer and inconsistent. Only studies with caries lesions as an end point should therefore be used for treatment recommendations and evidence-based guidelines.

TOPICAL APPLICATION OF ANTIBACTERIAL AGENTS

The most commonly suggested antiseptic agents to prevent and manage dental caries are CHX, povidine iodine, triclosan, and silver diamine fluoride (SDF). They all act on the protective side of the caries balance (**Fig. 2**).

CHX

CHX gluconate is effective against a wide variety of gram-negative and gram-positive organisms, aerobes, facultative anaerobes, and yeast. The use in general medicine is primarily for surgical scrub, hand rinse, and cleansing skin wounds. Within dentistry, CHX is the gold standard for plaque and gingivitis control and for irrigation during periodontal procedures.[9] Another common indication is temporary support of oral hygiene in medically compromised and disabled patients, including sick children. For oral use, CHX is available as rinsing solutions, gels, or dental varnishes at various concentrations (0.1%–40%; only 0.12% and 1% concentrations are available in the United States). The drug has a strong affinity to oral structures and the mechanism of action is 2-fold; at lower concentrations, CHX interferes with cell wall transportation and metabolic pathways, whereas higher concentrations cause precipitation of the intracellular cytoplasm. The bacterial population in plaque and saliva can be reduced by 80% immediately after a 0.2% CHX rinse. Long-term use of CHX mouth rinse does

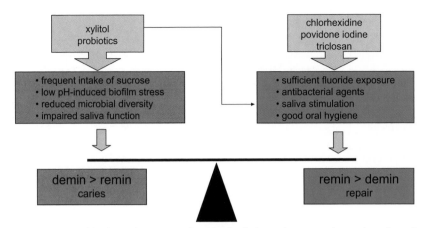

Fig. 2. Examples of biologic factors involved in the balance between de- and remineralization and the influence of some caries control measures. Xylitol and probiotics act mainly on the pathologic side to counteract the pH stress and maintain diversity, whereas the antiseptic agents work on the protective side.

not seem to confer any significant changes in bacterial resistance or overgrowth of potentially opportunistic organisms. The number of target bacteria in plaque, such as mutans streptococci, always returns to baseline within weeks or months after discontinuation of therapy. Extensive use of CHX for long periods can cause stained teeth, especially on resin restorations, and alter taste sensation.

The traditional indication for CHX treatment is caries control in caries-active individuals, and the best mode of professional treatment seems to be intensive treatments with gel in custom-made soft trays, 3 × 5 minutes for 2 consecutive days.[10] For home-care use, a 5-minute application once a day for 14 days may be preferred. Varnishes exert a slow release of CHX but must be reapplied at regular intervals. Detergents in toothpaste can inactivate CHX, and tooth brushing should therefore be separated from the agent by at least 2 hours. Although commonly used in Europe and Asia, no CHX formulation is approved for caries prevention in the United States.

CHX and Caries Prevention/Control

The first major prospective trial with CHX gel indicated an 85% reduction of caries in teenagers, with initially high counts (>10^6 cfu/mL) of salivary mutans streptococci.[11] Another successful approach for proximal caries control was to combine repeated CHX gel applications with professional interdental flossing.[12] A meta-analysis of all the early investigations revealed a prevented fraction of 46%,[13] but this figure was probably affected by publication bias because positive and novel findings are more likely to be published than negative. The initially successful findings with CHX regimes have not been confirmed in more recent trials conducted in situ or in high-risk children.[14–19] Consequently, later systematic reviews have resulted in more cautious conclusions, indicating a modest caries-preventive effect of around 10% to 26% (**Table 1**). Concerning CHX varnish, a recent review by Zhang and colleagues[20] concluded a moderate caries-inhibiting effect when varnish is applied every 3 to 4 months but the beneficial effect was questionable in low-caries populations. The findings in children are parallel with those in older adults; a recent study failed to show that regular rinsing with CHX could reduce root caries and preserve sound tooth structure in elderly people.[21]

Table 1
Prevented fraction[a] (PF) for various antimicrobial caries-preventive methods as extracted from meta-analysis (MA), systematic reviews (SR), or narrative reviews (NR)

Method	Publication Type	Number of Publications	Age Group	PF (%)	Year Ref no.
CHX agents	MA	8	School children	46	1996[13]
CHX agents	SR	7	All ages	26	2001[17]
CHX + fluoride	SR	6	All ages	26	2001[17]
CHX varnish, fissures	NR	5	School children	28	2004[18]
CHX varnish	SR	10	Children, young adults	10	2006[20]
CHX agents	NR	10[b]	All ages	Not reported	2008[22]
PI	NR	4	ECC[c]	20	2010[50]
SDF	SR	2	ECC	70	2009[31]
Xylitol	SR	6	School children	59	2008[49]
Xylitol products	NR	10[d]	All ages	35	2009[55]

[a] The difference in mean caries increments between the treatment and control groups expressed as a percentage of the mean increment in the control group.
[b] Based on published reviews.
[c] Early childhood caries.
[d] Published 2000–2008.

CHX rinses, gels, and varnishes have variable effects on mutans streptococci suppression and caries control. Because of the contradicting evidence, CHX rinses should not be recommended for primary caries prevention.[22] The evidence for gels and varnishes is mixed[20] but a small or modest anticaries effect in fissures and proximal surfaces in young permanent dentition is suggested. Lack of evidence based on statistical evaluations is not necessarily the same as lack of effect on the individual patient. A caries-active patient or a patient at risk may benefit from CHX applications as caries control provided that motivation and good compliance can be obtained. In such patients, the effect of the treatment should be monitored and verified through salivary tests.

Povidone Iodine

Povidone iodine (PI) is known as a powerful germicidal agent effective against a wide range of bacteria, viruses, fungi, protozoa, and spores. In medicine, PI is commonly used as skin disinfectant and for the treatment of wounds. A 10% solution can be used for topical oral applications and a moderate suppression of mutans streptococci in plaque and saliva is evident. PI has primarily been used in the United States to combat early childhood caries but the available studies are small and have contrasting findings. Although Lopez and colleagues[23,24] reported favorable results in Puerto Rican infants, other researchers have been unable to confirm an additional effect in adjunct to fluoride and extensive restorative procedures.[25,26] Thus, no firm conclusion on the efficacy of PI in preventing caries can be drawn, and restrictive use is further justified because PI may cause skin irritation and severe allergic reactions.

Triclosan

Triclosan is a synthetic broad-spectrum antimicrobial agent with antiviral and antifungal properties. The biocide acts by blocking the active site of an essential enzyme in the cell membrane synthesis and is commonly used in detergents, soaps, and surface decontaminants. Triclosan/copolymer added to fluoride toothpastes has been shown to reduce supragingival plaque and gingivitis in humans[27] but the anticaries potential does not seem to be enhanced in adults.[28,29] However, a recent study comparing a 2430 ppm fluoride toothpaste with and without triclosan/copolymer showed a significantly lower increment of root and crown caries after 3 years.[30] Although some concerns on bacterial resistance have been raised, the Scientific Committee on Consumer Products of the European Commission has stated that the use of triclosan in cosmetic products is safe.

SDF

Silver compounds have a long history in pediatric dentistry and have traditionally been used to halt rampant caries in young children (Howe solution). The rational is that silver salts effectively can kill bacteria and inhibit biofilm formation and stimulate dentine formation at Ag^+ concentrations exceeding 50 ppm. A recent systematic review by Rosenblatt and colleagues[31] examined the clinical evidence for SDF. These investigators identified 2 studies that reported a prevented fraction for caries arrest and caries prevention of 96% and 70%, respectively. Black staining was troublesome for 7% of the patients and a few experienced transient tissue irritations. The research on SDF is limited and it is unclear whether or not this historical therapy to arrest caries lesion progression has a place in modern practice. It may be useful as a low-cost alternative for secondary prevention for children in developing countries with limited access to dental care.

LIMITATIONS OF THE ANTIBACTERIAL APPROACH TO PREVENT CARIES

What is the reason for the limited outcome of the antibacterial measures taken for caries prevention and control? An easy answer would be that neither fluoride nor chemotherapeutics fully counteract or compensate the carbohydrate challenge and pH stress that are the key causes of caries. Caries is not a classic infectious disease that can be cured with 1 week of antibiotic treatment. Even extensive efforts to control the disease can fail, and genetic differences with respect to caries susceptibility may be overlooked.[32] A more complex answer may be found in recent insights concerning the functions of the oral biofilm. Caries-associated bacteria are sensitive to antibacterial agents in planktonic monocultures using traditional culturing techniques. However, the complex and diverse biofilm in the oral cavity, consisting of more than 900 different species, is characterized by an increased tolerance to antibacterial agents[33] and the effect in vivo may be short-term and transient. The reasons for this impaired efficacy are not fully known but factors such as inhibition of diffusion, bacterial cross-talk, reactions to stress, and upregulation of protein production are likely to play an important role. Another key question is whether or not it is advisable, or even realistic, to try to eradicate certain pathogenic strains from the biofilm. As mentioned earlier, caries is a result of an adaptation of the microbial community to environmental stress.[34] Various bacteria may act friendly or hostile, and oral health is associated with a diverse and balanced microbial community (microbial homeostasis) that is protective against invasions of pathogens. The ecological long-term strategy to combat oral diseases is therefore to restore the microbial balance rather than remove or kill selective pathogens, especially because the kill approach may create sites for rapid repopulation by pathogens.[35] Novel antibacterial and pH approaches to modify the oral biofilm diversity beneficially are emerging as an alternative to selective killing. Examples are replacement therapy with probiotics, and plant-derived agents and peptides regulating bacterial metabolism. Probiotics have advanced to human controlled caries trials and are further discussed later.

REPLACEMENT THERAPY AND PROBIOTICS

Defense through diversity means that bacteria associated with health take a place in the biofilm that otherwise would be occupied by a pathogen, and underabundant strains are promoted to maintain or reestablish the diversity. Probiotics (derived from the Greek *pro bios*, for life) are defined by the World Health Organization as "live microorganisms which when administered in adequate amounts confer a health benefit on the host." A regular intake of probiotics is classified as safe by food and drug agencies around the world,[36] but certain restrictiveness should be exercised for seriously ill patients with a depressed immunologic response, for example, those with the human immunodeficiency virus and leukemia. Probiotics are nonmodified human isolates from healthy individuals and most of them belong to the lactobacilli and bifidobacteria groups which are naturally present in the intestinal flora.

Mechanisms of Action

Despite intensive research over the years, detailed understanding of the mechanisms of action is still incomplete. Three main routes can be distinguished:

1. Probiotic bacteria compete for nutrients and binding sites in the biofilm.
2. When attached, probiotic bacteria can produce bacteriocins (eg, hydrogen peroxide and reuterin) that hamper and inhibit growth of a variety of bacteria.
3. Probiotic bacteria stimulate the specific and nonspecific immune response through activation of T cells and production of cytokines that mediates the inflammatory process.

Probiotics can thus influence the oral cavity and the caries balance locally and systemically: locally through a direct contact with the oral tissues and systemically (indirect) via the gastrointestinal tract. Studies have shown that probiotic bacteria can survive and grow in saliva, attach to the oral biofilm and coaggregate with caries-associated bacteria.[37,38] However, it is unlikely that a permanent colonization occurs. Therefore, regular consumption of probiotic products is needed to maintain the preventive and therapeutic levels. A daily intake of 1 to 2 dL of fluid (eg, yogurt) with about 10^8 live bacteria per mL is advocated. The corresponding recommendation for tablets and capsules is 2 pieces per day. As the composition of the biofilm in infants is immature, it has been suggested that an intake of probiotic bacteria early in life could lead to a permanent colonization, but there are still no studies of good quality with dental focus to support this assumption.

Effect on General Health and Caries Prevention

It is generally accepted that a daily intake of live lactobacilli and bifidobacteria reduces the risk of certain gastrointestinal problems.[39] In addition, a wide range of health effects have been suggested (eg, reduced susceptibility to infections, reduced prevalence of allergies and lactose intolerance). The strongest evidence for a therapeutic effect is related to infant diarrhea and for the management of diarrhea associated with treatment with broad-spectrum antibiotics.

There is fair evidence to suggest that a regular consumption of probiotic bacteria can lead to a significant reduction of mutans streptococci in saliva[40] without any significant increase in lactobacilli levels. Concerns have been raised that the introduction of homo- and hetero-fermentative lactobacilli could increase acid production in the biofilm but studies have shown that *Lactobacillus rhamnosus* and *L reuteri* have a low metabolic activity when exposed to sugars.[41] Probiotics in dairy products is an attractive combination from a cariological point of view because milk-derived products contain calcium, phosphate, and casein needed for remineralization. Many over-the-counter drinks and yogurts contain excessive amounts of added sugars and should therefore be avoided.

To date, there are 2 clinical trials that evaluate the effects of probiotics on caries development. In a Finnish study, preschool children were served milk containing *L rhamnosus* LGG over a period of 7 months, which reduced the risk for caries compared with a control group who received conventional milk.[42] A side effect was that significantly fewer upper respiratory infections were evident as well as a reduced need of antibiotics. A similar study was recently completed in northern Sweden in which preschool children at caries risk were served milk supplemented with a combination of *L rhamnosus* LB21 and 2.5 ppm of fluoride.[43] Caries increment was scored at the dentin level. After 21 months, the prevented fraction was 75% compared with a control group who received standard milk. Also in this project, a significantly diminished need for antibiotic prescriptions was shown as well as a lowered incidence of middle-ear infections. The use of probiotics is promising but the safety and clinical efficacy must be further established in controlled trials before any evidence-based regimens can be considered.

DIETARY CONTROL AND SUGAR SUBSTITUTES

The ecology of the biofilm can be beneficially modified by excluding fermentable carbohydrates, and especially sucrose, from the diet.[44] This seems far from realistic, however, with a current average sucrose consumption ranging between 40 and 60 kg per capita and year in industrialized countries. Furthermore, the effectiveness of dietary measures to prevent caries seems limited. Various sugar substitutes have therefore gained interest, and xylitol has emerged as the most powerful candidate among the polyols. Xylitol is a naturally occurring caloric 5-carbon sugar alcohol that is non-fermentable by oral bacteria and may influence the oral ecology through a chain of different antibacterial events[45]:

1) Xylitol hampers bacterial metabolism and diminishes the pH decrease in the dental plaque. The polyol is incorporated by oral bacteria with the fructose-specific phosphotransferase system and phosphorylated to xylitol-5-phosphate, which is a toxic end point. Only a few oral species can use this substance for energy production.
2) Xylitol reduces the volume and amount of supragingival plaque caused by a reduced production of extracellular polysaccharides and biofilm matrix.
3) Xylitol promotes the selection of xylitol-resistant mutans streptococci, which are believed to be less virulent and adhesive than xylitol-susceptible strains.
4) Xylitol exerts a stimulating effect on saliva secretion.

Collectively, these properties suggest that xylitol has a dual effect on the caries balance by decreasing the acid challenge on the pathologic side and by promoting remineralization through saliva stimulation on the protective side (see **Fig. 2**).

Evidence for Anticaries Effects

There are several reviews of the caries-preventive efficacy of xylitol but the conclusions differ in substantial ways. Whereas some investigators conclude that xylitol is superior to other polyols and has an important role in caries prevention,[46,47] others claim that the beneficial effects primarily are based on saliva stimulation.[48] The initial xylitol studies were field projects based on cohorts with remarkable results. For example, the pioneering landmark trial, the Turku Sugar Studies in 1975, presented an almost complete eradication of caries increment within 25 months after total sugar replacement. Later studies conducted in high-caries populations in developing countries even indicated that caries lesions could be reversed. Thus, when the results from the early controlled and observational studies were compiled, a caries-prevented fraction of 59% was reported.[49] A more cautious figure emerges when only data from the major controlled clinical trials from the present decade are taken into account.[50] Eight of the 10 reports included had results in favor of xylitol, although the difference between test and control groups was not always statistically significant. The mean prevented fraction was 35%. Few studies were placebo-controlled, however, and because comparisons with no-treatment groups have a tendency to overestimate the treatment effect it is likely that the true value is even lower. Nevertheless, a conservative conclusion from the recent trials is that a beneficial effect of xylitol on caries development in children and young adults cannot be excluded and the evidence is rated as fair. Few studies have been conducted in adults or elderly patients, which means that there is a lack of knowledge on the efficacy of xylitol regimes in those age groups.

Dose-Response

Xylitol is available in a wide range of commercial products such as toothpaste, chewing gums, slow-melting tablets, syrup, and candy. High single doses can result in osmotic diarrhea, which can be prevented by slow and stepwise introduction together with fractioned doses. Reports of adverse effects from the clinical trials are scarce, however, indicating that xylitol is well accepted by the patients. From recent studies it has become evident that a dose-response relationship exists and that the frequency of administration could affect the antibacterial outcome[51] and the minimum amount of xylitol needed for a beneficial effect on the biofilm is 5 to 6 g per day. Evidence-based clinical guidelines are presented in the following list. The clinical use of xylitol is recommended for children more than 4 years of age by several dental associations, including the American Academy of Pediatric Dentistry. The challenge of the dental professional is to advocate a convenient way to administrate xylitol in sufficient amounts, adjusted to age, but also realistic from an economical point of view.

Guidelines for patient-based caries management with xylitol-containing products

- Patients at caries risk could be recommended to use xylitol-containing products as a complement to the daily fluoride exposure.
- At least 5 g of xylitol per day is needed to optimize the beneficial effects on oral ecology.
- The daily intake should be divided into 3 to 4 doses, for example morning, noon, and evening. The exposure time should not be shorter than 5 to 10 minutes.
- Xylitol products that actively stimulate saliva secretion should be advocated.
- Recommended products should contain as much xylitol per unit as possible and with xylitol as the single sweetener.

Target Patients for Xylitol

A common recommendation is that xylitol-containing oral products should be included in the armamentarium for preventing caries in patients at high risk or in caries-active patients,[52] but there are few studies to support this. One recent randomized controlled trial included xylitol among other preventive measures in a 3-year intensive program for caries-active adolescents, with a focus on self-empower-ment and healthy behavior.[53] The program resulted in significantly less decay but the relative effect of the various components of the program remained unclear. A common problem with high-risk patients is that they have a tendency not to follow the protocol and the studies often suffer from poor compliance and high dropout rates. Other suggested target groups for xylitol-based interventions include caries-active preschool children and frail elderly patients as well as mentally and physically disabled patients.[50,54] Studies have also indicated that adolescents undergoing treatment with fixed orthodontic appliances may benefit from habitual intake of xylitol-containing lozenges or gums to reduce risk for white spot lesion development adjacent to the fixed appliances.[50] Xylitol-based interventions have also proved successful in clinical trials with the aim of diminishing and delaying the early transmission of mutans strep-tococci from highly colonized mothers to their offspring.[45]

SUMMARY

- Chair-side saliva diagnostics provide information on factors involved in the caries balance.
- There is incomplete evidence to support and recommend general topical appli-cations of antibacterial agents, such as CHX and PI, to prevent caries lesions. Antiseptic strategies may still have value in certain selected high-risk and caries-active patients, but definitive trials are needed.
- Emerging data suggest that regular consumption of probiotic bacteria can reduce mutans streptococci counts and caries risk, but many questions remain to be answered before any clinical recommendations can be given.
- There is a good body of evidence that xylitol has antibacterial properties that may alter the oral ecology and reduce caries risk, but the clinical evidence is rated as fair.
- Preventive programs should include as many complementary strategies as possible, especially when directed toward caries-active patients. Therefore, any antibacterial intervention should be combined with a fluoride program.

REFERENCES

1. Selwitz RH, Ismail AI, Pitts NB. Dental caries. Lancet 2007;369(9555):51–9.
2. Featherstone JD. The caries balance: the basis for caries management by risk assessment. Oral Health Prev Dent 2004;2(Suppl 1):259–64.
3. Marsh PD. Dental plaque as a biofilm: the significance of pH in health and caries. Compend Contin Educ Dent 2009;30(2):76–8, 80, 83–7.
4. The Swedish Council on Technology Assessment in Health Care. Caries – diag-nosis, risk assessment and non-invasive treatment. A systematic review. Summary and Conclusions. Report No 188. Stockholm (Sweden): The Swedish Council on Technology Assessment in Health Care; 2007. p. 15–29.
5. Tenovuo J. Salivary parameters of relevance for assessing caries activity in indi-viduals and populations. Community Dent Oral Epidemiol 1997;25(1):82–6.
6. Twetman S, Fontana M. Patient caries risk assessment. Monogr Oral Sci 2009;21:91–101.
7. Thenisch NL, Bachmann LM, Imfeld T, et al. Are mutans streptococci detected in preschool children a reliable predictive factor for dental caries risk? A systematic review. Caries Res 2006;40(5):366–74.

8. Ollila PS, Larmas MA. Long-term predictive value of salivary microbial diagnostic tests in children. Eur Arch Paediatr Dent 2008;9(1):25–30.
9. Gunsolley JC. A meta-analysis of six-month studies of antiplaque and antigingivitis agents. J Am Dent Assoc 2006;137(12):1649–57.
10. Emilson CG. Potential efficacy of chlorhexidine against mutans streptococci and human dental caries. J Dent Res 1994;73(3):682–91.
11. Zickert I, Emilson CG, Krasse B. Effect of caries preventive measures in children highly infected with the bacterium *Streptococcus mutans*. Arch Oral Biol 1982; 27(10):861–8.
12. Gisselsson H, Birkhed D, Björn AL. Effect of professional flossing with chlorhexidine gel on approximal caries in 12- to 15-year-old schoolchildren. Caries Res 1988;22(3):187–92.
13. van Rijkom HM, Truin GJ, van 't Hof MA. A meta-analysis of clinical studies on the caries-inhibiting effect of chlorhexidine treatment. J Dent Res 1996;75(2):790–5.
14. Ersin NK, Eden E, Eronat N, et al. Effectiveness of 2-year application of school-based chlorhexidine varnish, sodium fluoride gel, and dental health education programs in high-risk adolescents. Quintessence Int 2008;39(2):e45–51.
15. Petti S, Hausen H. Caries-preventive effect of chlorhexidine gel applications among high-risk children. Caries Res 2006;40(6):514–21.
16. van Strijp AJ, Gerardu VA, Buijs MJ, et al. Chlorhexidine efficacy in preventing lesion formation in enamel and dentine: an in situ study. Caries Res 2008;42(6):460–5.
17. Bader JD, Shugars DA, Bonito AJ. Systematic reviews of selected dental caries diagnostic and management methods. J Dent Educ 2001;65(10):960–8.
18. Twetman S. Antimicrobials in future caries control? A review with special reference to chlorhexidine treatment. Caries Res 2004;38(3):223–9.
19. Zhang Q, van 't Hof MA, Truin GJ, et al. Caries-inhibiting effect of chlorhexidine varnish in pits and fissures. J Dent Res 2006;85(5):469–72.
20. Zhang Q, van Palenstein Helderman WH, van't Hof MA, et al. Chlorhexidine varnish for preventing dental caries in children, adolescents and young adults: a systematic review. Eur J Oral Sci 2006;114(6):449–55.
21. Wyatt CC, Maupome G, Hujoel PP, et al. Chlorhexidine and preservation of sound tooth structure in older adults. A placebo-controlled trial. Caries Res 2007;41(2): 93–101.
22. Autio-Gold J. The role of chlorhexidine in caries prevention. Oper Dent 2008; 33(6):710–6.
23. Lopez L, Berkowitz R, Zlotnik H, et al. Topical antimicrobial therapy in the prevention of early childhood caries. Pediatr Dent 1999;21(1):9–11.
24. Lopez L, Berkowitz R, Spiekerman C, et al. Topical antimicrobial therapy in the prevention of early childhood caries: a follow-up report. Pediatr Dent 2002; 24(3):204–6.
25. Xu X, Li JY, Zhou XD, et al. Randomized controlled clinical trial on the evaluation of bacteriostatic and cariostatic effects of a novel povidone-iodine/fluoride foam in children with high caries risk. Quintessence Int 2009;40(3):215–23.
26. Zhan L, Featherstone JD, Gansky SA, et al. Antibacterial treatment needed for severe early childhood caries. J Public Health Dent 2006;66(3):174–9.
27. Gaffar A, Afflitto J, Nabi N. Chemical agents for the control of plaque and plaque microflora: an overview. Eur J Oral Sci 1997;105(5 Pt2):502–7.
28. Feller RP, Kiger RD, Triol CW, et al. Comparison of the clinical anticaries efficacy of an 1100 NaF silica-based dentifrice containing triclosan and a copolymer to an 1100 NaF silica-based dentifrice without those additional agents: a study on adults in California. J Clin Dent 1996;7(4):85–9.

29. Mann J, Karniel C, Triol CW, et al. Comparison of the clinical anticaries efficacy of a 1500 NaF silica-based dentifrice containing triclosan and a copolymer to a 1500 NaF silica-based dentifrice without those additional agents: a study on adults in Israel. J Clin Dent 1996;7(4):90–5.

30. Vered Y, Zini A, Mann J, et al. Comparison of a dentifrice containing 0.243% sodium fluoride, 0.3% triclosan, and 2.0% copolymer in a silica base, and a dentifrice containing 0.243% sodium fluoride in a silica base: a three-year clinical trial of root caries and dental crowns among adults. J Clin Dent 2009;20(2):62–5.

31. Rosenblatt A, Stamford TC, Niederman R. Silver diamine fluoride: a caries "silver-fluoride bullet". J Dent Res 2009;88(2):116–25.

32. Bretz WA, Corby PM, Schork NJ, et al. Longitudinal analysis of heritability for dental caries traits. J Dent Res 2005;84(11):1047–51.

33. Gilbert P, Das J, Foley I. Biofilm susceptibility to antimicrobials. Adv Dent Res 1997;11(1):160–7.

34. Li Y, Ge Y, Saxena D, et al. Genetic profiling of the oral microbiota associated with severe early-childhood caries. J Clin Microbiol 2007;45(1):81–7.

35. He X, Lux R, Kuramitsu HK, et al. Achieving probiotic effects via modulating oral microbial ecology. Adv Dent Res 2009;21:53–6.

36. de Vrese M, Schrezenmeier L. Probiotics, prebiotics and synbiotics. Adv Biochem Eng Biotechnol 2008;111:1–66.

37. Haukioja A, Yli-Knuuttila H, Loimaranta V, et al. Oral adhesion and survival of probiotic and other lactobacilli and bifidobacteria in vitro. Oral Microbiol Immunol 2006;21(5):326–32.

38. Twetman L, Larsen U, Fiehn NE, et al. Coaggregation between probiotic bacteria and caries-associated strains: an in vitro study. Acta Odontol Scand 2009;67(5):284–8.

39. Doron S, Gorbach SL. Probiotics: their role in the treatment and prevention of disease. Expert Rev Anti Infect Ther 2006;4(2):261–75.

40. Twetman S, Stecksén-Blicks C. Probiotics and oral health effects in children. Int J Paediatr Dent 2008;18(1):3–10.

41. Hedberg M, Hasslöf P, Sjöström I, et al. Sugar fermentation in probiotic bacteria–an in vitro study. Oral Microbiol Immunol 2008;23(6):482–5.

42. Näse L, Hatakka K, Savilahti E, et al. Effect of long term consumption of a probiotic bacterium, Lactobacillus rhamnosus GG, in milk on dental caries and caries risk in children. Caries Res 2001;35(6):412–20.

43. Stecksén-Blicks C, Sjöström I, Twetman S. Effect of long-term consumption of milk supplemented with probiotic lactobacilli and fluoride on dental caries and general health in preschool children: a cluster-randomized study. Caries Res 2009;43(5):374–81.

44. Beighton D. Can the ecology of the dental biofilm be beneficially altered? Adv Dent Res 2009;21:69–73.

45. Söderling EM. Xylitol, mutans streptococci, and dental plaque. Adv Dent Res 2009;21:74–8.

46. Burt BA. The use of sorbitol- and xylitol-sweetened chewing gum in caries control. J Am Dent Assoc 2006;137(2):190–6.

47. Maguire A, Rugg-Gunn A. Xylitol and caries prevention – is it a magical bullet? Braz Dent J 2003;194(8):429–36.

48. Mickenautsch S, Leal SC, Yengopal, et al. Sugar-free chewing gums and dental caries – a systematic review. J Appl Oral Sci 2007;15(2):83–8.

49. Deshpande A, Jadad AR. The impact of polyol-containing chewing gums on dental caries: a systematic review of original randomized controlled trials and observational studies. J Am Dent Assoc 2008;139(12):1602–4.

50. Twetman S. Current controversies–is there merit? Adv Dent Res 2009;21:48–52.
51. Milgrom P, Ly KA, Rothen M. Xylitol and its vehicles for public health needs. Adv Dent Res 2009;21:44–7.
52. Ly KA, Milgrom P, Rothen M. Xylitol, sweeteners and dental caries. Pediatr Dent 2006;28(2):154–63.
53. Hausen H, Seppä L, Poutanen R, et al. Non-invasive control of dental caries in children with active initial lesions. A randomized clinical trial. Caries Res 2007; 41(5):384–91.
54. Milgrom P, Zero DT, Tanzer JM. An examination of the advances in science and technology of prevention of tooth decay in young children since the Surgeon General's Report on Oral Health. Acad Pediatr 2009;9(6):404–9.
55. Twetman S. Antibacterial agents for prevention and therapy of early childhood caries. Oralprophylaxe & Kinderzahnheilkunde 2010;32, in press.

Clinical Threshold for Carious Tissue Removal

Edwina A.M. Kidd, BDS, FDSRCS, PhD, DSc Med*

KEYWORDS

- Caries removal • Operative dentistry • Stepwise excavation
- Caries microbiology • Incomplete caries removal

"The complete divorcement of dental practice from the studies of the pathology of dental caries, that existed in the past, is an anomaly in science that should not continue. It has the apparent tendency to make dentists mechanics only."

Thus wrote GV Black in his textbook of operative dentistry in 1908.[1] This seminal text was in two volumes, and Volume 1 was entirely devoted to the pathology of the hard tissues of the teeth; his suggestions for caries management were based on his observations of the disease process.

Unfortunately, in the intervening century, something went strangely wrong, because in many dental schools the science of cariology and the technicalities of operative dentistry were taught and researched separately. Generations of students passed through operative technique courses and phantom head rooms restoring caries-free natural teeth or, even worse, plastic counterfeits. The eventual appearance of demineralized tissue in living patients on the clinic could be a considerable inconvenience, ruining stereotyped outline forms and preconceptions of appropriate depths, widths, and angles.[2]

Current practice in caries removal cuts back enamel to expose softened infected dentin. The enamel–dentin junction is instrumented further until it is hard and in some countries until it is also stain-free. Over the pulpal surface, softened, demineralized dentin is scooped away with sharp small spoons called excavators. The point of terminating excavation varies according to the country, dental school, the individual teacher's idiosyncrasy, and the presumed proximity of the softened tissue to the pulp. This article assembles the biologic evidence behind what needs to be removed and will, rather uncomfortably, challenge conventional teaching. Some will consider these suggestions to be heresy, while others may have been working in this way for years and will wonder what all the fuss is about.

Kings College London, England, UK
* 57 Langley Avenue, Surbiton, Surrey, KT6 6QR, England, UK.
E-mail address: thelittletons@aol.co.uk

Dent Clin N Am 54 (2010) 541–549
doi:10.1016/j.cden.2010.03.001
0011-8532/10/$ – see front matter © 2010 Elsevier Inc. All rights reserved.

dental.theclinics.com

WHAT IS CARIES?

It is perhaps unfortunate that the word caries is used to describe both the caries process and the caries lesion. The caries process occurs in the biofilm, a community of microorganisms with a collective physiology that respond to the environment at the site. The biofilm is always metabolically active with minute fluctuations in pH. The result may be nothing to see or there may be a net loss of mineral, leading to a caries lesion that can be seen. Thus, caries the process occurs in the biofilm, and the interaction of the biofilm with the tooth surface may result in the formation of caries the lesion, the consequence or reflection of the process.

CARIES CONTROL BY NONOPERATIVE TREATMENTS

Wherever a patient can access and disturb the biofilm with a fluoride-containing dentifrice, a filling is not needed.[3] This simple cleaning measure will control caries lesion progression. No fillings are required in the following circumstances:

White spot lesions including those on occlusal surfaces[1,4]

Approximal caries lesions where the lesion is confined to the enamel, or just into dentin on bitewing radiograph. These lesions are unlikely to be cavitated in contemporary populations and should be given a chance to arrest with nonoperative treatments[3]

Root surface lesions accessible to cleaning, both cavitated and noncavitated[5]

Recurrent caries lesions adjacent to fillings, uncavitated or cavitated but cleansable, also do not require restorations. Amalgam fillings should not be replaced simply because of ditching and staining around them. Mild ditching, that a periodontal probe will not enter, and staining around a restoration are poor predictors of infected dentin beneath the restoration[6]

Large cavitated lesions where overhanging enamel has been removed by the dentist, or has fractured away, are also cleansable and can be arrested by cleaning alone. This is a clinical observation. The author does not know of a clinical study that has addressed this in a controlled manner.

WHEN IS A FILLING NEEDED TO CONTROL CARIES?

A cavitated lesion, where the patient cannot access the biofilm with a toothbrush, is likely to progress and requires restoration as part of caries lesion control.[3] Put simply, the filling restores the integrity of the tooth surface and allows the patient to clean again. Thus, from a cariological point of view, restoring the tooth is part of plaque control.

Fillings are required in the following circumstances:

Cavitated occlusal lesions, (codes 3 or higher ICDAS II, see the article by Braga and colleagues elsewhere in this issue for further exploration of this topic); these are likely to be visible in dentine on a bitewing radiograph[7,8]

Cavitated approximal lesions; these are clearly into dentin on a bitewing radiograph.[3]

OBJECTIVES OF RESTORATION FROM A CARIOLOGICAL POINT OF VIEW

Caries removal and restoration should:

Arrest caries lesion progression

Provide an adequate base for the restorative material

Produce a filling that the patient can clean.

The advent of adhesive restorative materials was particularly exciting, because whereas amalgam could be regarded as a plug in a hole, bonded adhesive materials might be capable of improving cavity seal and even giving back some strength to tooth tissue undermined by demineralization. Good cavity seal is thought to be of great import, because it is leakage of bacteria that potentially damages a vital pulp.[9] Supporting tooth tissue undermined by demineralization may allow preparations to be much more conservative, preserving tissue that would have to be removed without the strengthening effect of the adhesive material.[10]

AN OLD ARGUMENT

Discussions on how much demineralized tissue must be removed before restoration are hardly new. One can go back 150 years to Tomes[11] writing in 1859:

"It is better that a layer of discoloured dentine should be allowed to remain for the protection of the pulp rather than run the risk of sacrificing the tooth."

Black,[12] however, did not agree for he wrote in 1908

"...it will often be a question of whether or not the pulp will be exposed when all decayed dentin overlaying it is removed....it is better to expose the pulp of a tooth than to leave it covered only with softened dentin."

This article now focuses on the biologic arguments for and against vigorous caries removal before examining the research evidence on the consequences of incomplete caries removal.

PULPO–DENTINAL REACTIONS TO DENTAL CARIES

Dentin is a vital, cellular tissue, containing the cellular processes of the odontoblasts. Thus dentin and pulp must be considered together. The ecological catastrophe in the biofilm, which is the caries disease process, is an assault on this vital tissue that is capable of defending itself. In 1967, Massler distilled current scientific knowledge on this matter including describing his own research performed over a period of 11 years on more than 800 human teeth.[13] His sense of frustration at some of his colleagues jumps from the page:

"It is somewhat disturbing to the biologically orientated clinical teacher to witness the overly focused attention of some dentists upon the operative and restorative phases of dentistry, the 'drilling and filling' of teeth, to the neglect of the disease process which caused the lesion (cariology) and the preoperative treatment of the wounded tooth–bone."

A combination of defense and degenerative reactions characterizes the caries lesion in the pulpo–dentinal complex. Massler's particular contribution was to point out how essential it is to differentiate active from arrested lesions if one is to make any sense of the biologic reactions. From this, a logical management follows. This seeks to convert an active lesion into an inactive or arrested lesion, thus aiding the defense and healing processes in dentin and pulp before restorative procedures are attempted.

Massler showed that under an active lesion, the dentinal tubules were permeable, whereas under arrested lesions, there were sclerotic zones in the dentin that were impermeable to dyes and isotopes.[13] He pointed out that the plugging of the tubules forms a very effective barrier against further penetration of toxic materials toward the pulp. Thus it would be biologically crazy to damage this area by attacking it with a bur.

Massler described an active lesion as one characterized by an active bacterial colony on the surface (the infected layer) and a very wide layer of demineralized dentin beneath, containing few pathogenic microorganisms (the affected dentin). Massler subsequently pointed out that most lesions found clinically were a combination of active and arrested lesions. At the periphery of the lesion, an active lesion is often spreading under the overhanging enamel, along the enamel–dentin junction, while the central, more easily cleaned area is hard and partially remineralized. Thus, as stated at the beginning of this article, the lesion reflects the activity in the overlying biofilm.

CAN AND SHOULD INFECTED DENTIN BE REMOVED?

If the biofilm at the tooth surface drives the caries lesion, all that must be removed to arrest the lesion is the biofilm. Supposing a clinician disagrees with this interpretation and wishes to remove all the infected dentin, can this be achieved? The answer is to this question is that it is not possible. Shovelton's review of 1968[14] showed that softening of dentin generally precedes the organisms responsible for it, but a few organisms will remain even if all the soft dentin is removed.

CONVENTIONAL CARIES REMOVAL

The most commonly used criterion for the removal of infected dentin is to scoop out all the soft stuff with an excavator. At the enamel–dentin junction, some schools teach the area should be made stain-free as well as hard; others just say hard and ignore the stain. Because staining is an unreliable guide to the level of infection of the dentin, and because a few bacteria will remain whatever approach is adopted, leaving stain seems more conservative.[15]

Over the pulpal surface, stained dentin should remain so long as it is reasonably hard. Provided a tooth is symptomless and responds as vital to pulp testing, vigorous excavation over the pulpal surface seems positively contraindicated once the cavity floor is reasonably firm. The student, however, will find that teachers do not agree on what constitutes reasonably firm. The subjectivity of these assessments led to the development by Fusayama[16,17] of red dyes to be used clinically to differentiate infected from affected dentin. Infected dentin was shown to be an irreversibly damaged layer, while affected dentin was the inner, remineralizable zone. The same author tentatively suggested the dye staining front coincided with the bacterial invasion front.

Thus, in theory, this dye could be used to identify the carious tissue that is infected with bacteria and thus needs to be excavated. Subsequently, several studies[18–20] showed the dye does not necessarily discriminate infected tissue and use of the dye could lead to overpreparation of cavities, encouraging removal of excess tissue at the enamel–dentin junction[20] and removal of sclerotic and reparative dentin over the pulpal surface.[21]

ULTRACONSERVATIVE CARIES REMOVAL

Thus far, this article has questioned the biologic basis for contemporary caries removal, which seeks to remove most infected demineralized dentin. Is this appropriate with the present knowledge about the disease and the way in which lesions progress? What would happen if most of the infected dentin were left and a restoration placed? Would the caries process arrest? There is much evidence to answer this question from:

Studies placing fissure sealants over carious dentin
Stepwise excavation studies
Studies where a final restoration was placed following incomplete caries removal

Randomized clinical trials comparing conventional and ultraconservative caries removal.

FISSURE SEALANT STUDIES

Several studies have examined the consequences of sealing over carious dentin.[22-30] All studies bar one[30] were prospective, and in many there were unsealed control lesions. Caries lesion activity was assessed in several ways, including clinical observation, clinical and radiographic lesion depth measurement, and microbiological sampling. Observation periods varied from 2 weeks to 5 years.

Some uniform themes emerge[2]:

Sealed lesions appeared to arrest clinically and radiographically
Microorganisms were eliminated or decreased with time
There was no pulpitis in sealed teeth
Lesions progressed where sealants were lost or in unsealed control teeth.

The study by Weerheijm and colleagues[30] is an interesting outlier. She accessed demineralized tissue in teeth with radiographic lesions in dentin under intact sealants. Cariogenic organisms were found in 50% of the teeth, and the dentin was often soft and moist, apparently indicating lesion activity.

STEPWISE EXCAVATION STUDIES

In stepwise excavation, only part of the soft dentin caries is removed at the first visit during the acute phase of caries progression.[31-45] The cavity is restored and reopened after a period of weeks. Further excavation then is performed before a definitive restoration. The objective of the exercise is to arrest lesion progression and allow the formation of reparative dentin, making pulpal exposure less likely in vital teeth with deep carious lesions but no symptoms of irreversible pulpitis.

The procedure has been investigated scientifically for over 30 years.[2] These studies have involved baseline investigation of carious dentin and then a reanalysis after a period of sealing. Collectively these studies tell much about the consequences of sealing infected dentin in teeth.

Most of the studies are done in permanent teeth with deep lesions, although some studies have involved deciduous teeth.[31,33-35] There are often no controls. The amount of dentin removed at the first visit varies greatly from only access to carious dentin to removing the bulk of the carious dentin. The restorative materials are also very variable, including calcium hydroxide, zinc oxide and eugenol, amalgam, glass ionomer cement, and composite resin. Times to re-entry can be as short as 3 weeks or as long as 2 years.

Caries lesion activity has been assessed clinically, radiographically, and often by microbiological examination at the original visit and on re-entry.

Despite these very different methodologies, several themes emerge:

Clinical success is high, exposure usually avoided in the stepwise group, and there are rarely symptoms between visits. On the other hand, exposure is common in control, conventionally excavated lesions
The dentin often is altered on re-entry, being dryer, harder, and darker
Microbiological monitoring indicates substantial reductions in cultivable flora, although some microorganisms may survive
Several studies suggest the organisms have altered on re-entry to a less cariogenic flora.[42-44] Biologically this is entirely logical, because the supply of nutrients will

diminish. Not only are the organisms cut off from the oral environment, they are cut off from nutrients from the pulpal side also by tubular sclerosis and reparative dentin. They are in a stressful environment and adapt accordingly. One study even showed the flora on re-entry to be identical in the fully excavated control teeth and the teeth where soft, heavily infected dentin was left.[45] Collectively, these studies seem to put the final nail in the coffin of excavating demineralized dentin because it is infected. The few microorganisms that survive seem opportunistic squatters adapted to their new environment.

WHY RE-ENTER?

It is only logical to question whether re-entry is needed. The final excavation allows the dentist to be sure there is no exposure, but it is unlikely to alter the microbiology. Not re-entering is the basis of the indirect pulp capping technique.[46–48] The difference in caries removal between the two techniques is the amount of soft dentin removed. In indirect pulp capping the dentist attempts to remove as much as possible, and because there is no way of knowing the proximity of the pulp, this is a fine and difficult judgment. No such worry exists in stepwise excavation.

STUDIES WHERE THE FINAL RESTORATION WAS PLACED OVER SOFT DENTIN

Two studies selected less advanced lesions and did not re-enter to remove the remaining soft dentin in the treatment groups. The work of Ribero and colleagues[49] (1999) on deciduous teeth concluded that the clinical performance of the restorations was not adversely affected by the incomplete caries removal after a year. The study by Mertz-Fairhurst and colleagues[50] (1998) was remarkable for a 10-year follow-up of occlusal restorations in permanent teeth placed over moist, soft, infected dentin left both at the enamel–dentin junction and over the pulp. Remarkably, half the patients were still available for recall after 10 years. Lesion progression was arrested, and there were no more clinical failures in this group than in the control groups with conventional caries removal, although it is not known if this observation would have changed if all the patients had been available for recall.

Finally a randomized controlled clinical trial of the Hall technique of stainless steel crowns on deciduous teeth must be added to the evidence.[51] In this technique, primary molar teeth with caries lesions affecting two or more surfaces are restored with a preformed stainless steel crown. Unlike the traditionally taught technique, however, no caries removal takes place and no tooth preparation is performed. The crown simply is filled with a glass ionomer cement and placed on the tooth with either finger pressure or the child's occlusal force. The study was performed in general practice, and the control restorations were conventionally placed fillings. Results at 2 years showed only 2% of teeth with pulpal pathology in the Hall group compared with 15% in the conventionally restored group. Loss of restoration or caries lesion progression occurred in 5% of the Hall group but in 46% if the control group. When children and care givers were asked at placement which technique they preferred, the Hall technique was favored by most.

SYSTEMATIC REVIEW; COMPLETE VERSUS ULTRACONSERVATIVE REMOVAL OF DECAYED TISSUE

The included papers in this study were two stepwise excavation studies, one on permanent teeth and one on deciduous teeth and two studies where caries was sealed permanently into teeth.[52] Several conclusions were drawn:

Partial caries removal in symptomless, primary or permanent teeth reduces the risk of pulpal exposure

No detriment to the patient in terms of pulpal symptoms was found

Partial caries removal would appear preferable in the deep lesion to reduce the risk of carious exposure

There is insufficient evidence to know whether it is necessary to re-enter and excavate further in the stepwise excavation technique, but studies that did not re-enter reported no adverse consequences

There is a need for further randomized control clinical investigations of the need to remove demineralized tissue before restoring teeth. In particular the use of the technique in approximal lesions needs investigation, and the possibility of an adverse effect on the filling material should be studied. For instance, would a composite restoration placed on soft dentin be more liable to fracture?

REFERENCES

1. Black GV. Operative dentistry, vol. 1. Pathology of the hard tissues of the teeth. Chicago (IL): Medico-Dental Publishing Company; 1908.
2. Kidd EAM, Bjorndal L, Beighton D, et al. Caries removal and the pulpo–dentinal complex. In: Fejerskov O, Kidd EAM, editors. Dental caries: the disease and its clinical management. 2nd edition. Oxford (UK): Blackwell Munksgaard; 2008. p. 368–83.
3. Kidd EAM, van Amerongen JP, van Amerongen WE. The role of operative dentistrry in caries control. In: Fejerskov O, Kidd EAM, editors. Dental caries: the disease and its clinical management. 2nd edition. Oxford (UK): Blackwell Munksgaard; 2008. p. 356–65.
4. Carvalho JC, Thylstrup A, Ekstrand K. Results after 3 years nonoperative occlusal caries treatment of erupting carious first molars. Community Dent Oral Epidemiol 1992;20:187–92.
5. Nyvad B, Fejerskov O. Active root surface caries converted into inactive caries as a response to oral hygiene. Scand J Dent Res 1986;94:281–4.
6. Kidd EAM, Joyston-Bechal S, Beighton D. Marginal ditching and staining as a predictor of secondary caries around amalgam restorations: a clinical and microbiological study. J Dent Res 1995;74:1206–11.
7. Ricketts DN, Kidd EA, Beighton D. Operative and microbiological validation of visual, radiographic, and electronic diagnosis of occlusal caries in noncavitated teeth judged to be in need of operative care. Br Dent J 1995;179:214–20.
8. Ricketts DN, Ekstrand KR, Kidd EA, et al. Relating visual and radiographic ranked scoring systems for occlusal caries detection to histological and microbiological evidence. Oper Dent 2002;27:231–7.
9. Bergenholtz G. Bacterial leakage around dental restorations—impact on the pulp. In: Anusavich KJ, editor. Quality evaluation of dental restorations; criteria for placement and replacement. Chicago (IL): Quintessence; 1989. p. 243–52.
10. van Amerongen JP, van Amerongen WE, Watson TM, et al. Restoring the tooth: the seal is the deal. In: Fejerskov O, Kidd EAM, editors. Dental caries; the disease and its clinical management. 2nd edition. Oxford (UK): Blackwell Munksgaard; 2008. p. 386–425.
11. Tomes J. A system of dental surgery. London (UK): John Churchill; 1859.
12. Black GV. Operative dentistry, vol. 11. The technical procedures in filling teeth. Chicago (IL): Medico-Dental Publishing Company; 1908.
13. Massler M. Pulpal reactions to dental caries. Int Dent J 1967;17:441–60.
14. Shovelton DS. A study of deep carious dentine. Int Dent J 1968;18:392–405.

15. Kidd EAM, Ricketts D, Beighton D. Criteria for caries removal at the enamel–dentine junction: a clinical and microbiological study. Br Dent J 1996;180:287–91.
16. Fusayama T, Terachima S. Differentiation of two layers of carious dentin by staining. J Dent Res 1972;51:866.
17. Fusayama T. Two layers of carious dentin: diagnosis and treatment. Oper Dent 1979;4:63–70.
18. Boston DW, Graver HT. Histological study of an acid red caries-disclosing dye. Oper Dent 1989;14:186–92.
19. Anderson MH, Loesch WJ, Charbeneau GT. Bacteriologic study of a basic fuchsin caries- disclosing dye. J Prosthet Dent 1985;54:51–5.
20. Kidd EAM, Joyston-Bechal S, Beighton D. The use of a caries detector dye during cavity preparation: a microbiological assessment. Br Dent J 1993;174:245–8.
21. Yip HK, Stevenson AG, Beeley JA. The specificity of caries detector dyes in cavity preparation. Br Dent J 1994;176:417–21.
22. Jeronimus DJ, Till MJ, Sveen OB. Reduced viability of microorganisms under dental sealants. J Dent Child 1975;42:275–80.
23. Handelman SL, Wahsburn F, Wopperer P. Two-year report of sealant effect on bacteria in dental caries. J Am Dent Assoc 1976;93:967–70.
24. Going RE, Loesch WJ, Granger DA, et al. The viability of microorganisms in carious lesions four years after covering with a fissure sealant. J Am Dent Assoc 1978;97:455–62.
25. Mertz-Fairhurst EJ, Schuster GS, Williams JE, et al. Clinical progress of sealed and unsealed caries. 1. Depth changes and bacterial counts. J Prosthet Dent 1979;42:521–6.
26. Mertz-Fairhurst EJ, Schuster GS, Williams JE, et al. Clinical progress of sealed and unsealed caries. 11. Standardized radiographs and clinical observations. J Prosthet Dent 1979;42:633–7.
27. Jenson OE, Handelman SL. Effect of an autopolymerizing sealant on viability of microflora in occlusal dental caries. Scand J Dent Res 1980;88:382–8.
28. Handelman SL, Leverette DH, Solomon ES, et al. Radiographic evaluation of the sealing of occlusal caries. Community Dent Oral Epidemiol 1981;9:256–9.
29. Mertz-Fairhurst EJ, Schuster GS, Fisrhurst CW. Arresting caries by sealants: results of a clinical study. J Am Dent Assoc 1986;112:194–8.
30. Weerheijm KL, de Soet JJ, van Amerongen WE, et al. Sealing of occlusal caries lesions: an alternative for curative treatment? J Dent Child 1992;59:263–8.
31. Law DA, Lewis TM. The effect of calcium hydroxide on deep carious lesions. Oral Surg Oral Med Oral Pathol 1961;14:1130–7.
32. Schouboe T, MacDonald JB. Prolonged viability of organisms sealed in dental caries. Arch Oral Biol 1962;7:525–6.
33. King JB, Crawford JJ, Lindahl RL. Indirect pulp capping: a bacteriologic study of deep carious dentin in human teeth. Oral Surg Oral Med Oral Pathol 1965;20:663–71.
34. Kerkhove BC, Herman SC, Klein AI, et al. A clinical and television densitometric evaluation of the indirect pulp capping technique. J Dent Child 1967;34:192–201.
35. Magnusson BO, Sundell SO. Stepwise excavation of deep carious lesions in primary molars. J Int Assoc Dent Child 1997;8:36–40.
36. Weerheijm KL, de Soet JJ, van Amerongen WE, et al. The effect of glass ionomer cement on carious dentin. Caries Res 1993;27:417–23.
37. Leskell E, Ridell K, Cvek M, et al. Pulp exposure after stepwise versus direct complete excavation of deep carious lesions in young posterior permanent teeth. Endod Dent Traumatol 1996;12:192–6.

38. Kreulen CM, de Soet JJ, Weerheijm KI, et al. In vivo cariostatic effect of resin modified cement and amalgam on dentine. Caries Res 1997;31:384–9.
39. Weerheijm KL, Kreulen CM, de Soet JJ, et al. Bacterial counts in carious dentine under restorations; 2-year in vivo effects. Caries Res 1999;33:130–4.
40. Bjorndal L, Larson T, Thylstrup A. A clinical and microbiological study of deep carious lesions during stepwise excavation using long treatment intervals. Caries Res 1997;31:717–36.
41. Bjorndal L, Thylstrup A. A practice-based study of stepwise excavation of deep carious lesions in permanent teeth: a 1-year follow up study. Community Dent Oral Epidemiol 1998;26:122–8.
42. Bjorndal L, Larson T. Changes in the cultivable flora in deep carious lesions following a stepwise excavation procedure. Caries Res 2000;34:502–8.
43. Maltz M, de Oliveira EF, Fontanella V, et al. A clinical, microbiologic, and radiographic study of deep caries lesions after incomplete caries removal. Quintessence Int 2002;33:151–9.
44. Paddick JS, Brailsford SR, Kidd EAM, et al. Phenotypic and genotypic selection of microbiota surviving under dental restorations. Appl Environ Microbiol 2005;71:2467–72.
45. Lula EC, Monteiro-Neto, Alves CM, et al. Microbiological analysis after complete or partial removal of carious dentin in primary teeth: a randomized clinical trial. Caries Res 2009;43:354–8.
46. Prader E. Conservative treatment of the floor of the carious cavity—carious dentine near the pulp. Int Dent J 1958;8:627–38.
47. Eidelman E, Finn SB, Koulourides T. Remineralization of carious dentin treated with calcium hydroxide. J Dent Child 1965;32:218–25.
48. Hilton TJ, Summit JB. Pulpal considerations. In: Summitt JB, Robbins JW, Schwartz RS, editors. Operative dentistry. Chicago (IL): Quintessence; 2000. p. 101–23.
49. Ribeiro CC, Baratieri LN, Perdigao J, et al. A clinical, radiographic, and scanning electron microscope evaluation of adhesive restorations on carious dentin in primary teeth. Quintessence Int 1999;30:591–9.
50. Mertz-Fairhurst E, Curtis JW, Ergle JW, et al. Ultraconservative and cariostatic sealed restorations: results at year 10. J Am Dent Assoc 1998;129:55–66.
51. Innes NP, Evans DJ, Stirrips DR. The Hall technique: a randomized controlled clinical trial of a novel method of managing carious primary molars in general dental practice: acceptability of the technique and outcomes at 23 months. BMC Oral Health 2007;7:18.
52. Ricketts DN, Kidd EA, Innes N, et al. Complete or ultraconservative removal of decayed tissue in unfilled teeth. Cochrane Database Syst Rev 2006;(3):CD003808.

Glass-Ionomer Cements as Restorative and Preventive Materials

Hien Ngo, BDS, MDS, PhD, FADI, FICD, FPFA

KEYWORDS

- Glass-ionomer cement • Therapeutic coating
- Internal remineralisation • Caries

This article will focus on glass-ionomer cement (GIC) and its role in the clinical management of caries. It begins with a brief description of GIC, the mechanism of fluoride release and ion exchange, the interaction between GIC and the external environment, and finally the ion exchange between GIC and the tooth at the internal interface. The importance of GIC, as a tool, in caries management, in minimal intervention dentistry, and Caries Management by Risk Assessment (CAMBRA) also will be highlighted.

The philosophy of minimal intervention density (MI) and the CAMBRA approach is gaining popularity worldwide as both integrate the new understanding that caries is a biofilm-related, multifactorial and lifestyle-associated bi-directional disease. There is now an acceptance that to manage caries disease effectively, it is important to move from the surgical approach to a combined surgical—medical approach, with special focus on engaging patients in changing their lifestyle. The following statement is a consensus of 165 experts, comprising of clinicians, scientists, educators, and health service managers from 15 countries, who gathered in Bangkok for a consultative meeting to discuss the MI philosophy (personal communication, 2009):

> "The current surgical model of caries management does not fully address the multi-factorial nature of dental caries. This model often results in unnecessary removal of tooth structure, can impact negatively on general health and quality of life and can impose substantial cost."

Glass-ionomer cement (GIC) is an important tool in the fight against caries. It can be thought of as a reservoir of fluoride and other ions in the oral cavity, a mechanical barrier that protects the tooth surface against bacteria; most importantly, it can provide a long-lasting seal under the most challenging clinical circumstances.

General Dental Practice, School of Dentistry, The University of Queensland, 200 Turbot Street, Brisbane, QLD 4000, Australia
E-mail address: h.ngo@uq.edu.au

Dent Clin N Am 54 (2010) 551–563
doi:10.1016/j.cden.2010.04.001
0011-8532/10/$ – see front matter © 2010 Published by Elsevier Inc.

dental.theclinics.com

GIC is very versatile. It may be utilized as a definitive restorative material, a preparation liner, a restorative base material, a luting cement, or a fissure sealant. Recently, it was suggested that GIC also could be useful in the preventive arena as therapeutic coating. This new terminology is utilized to describe a material that can be painted on a susceptible surface and form a long-lasting coat to protect, both mechanically and chemically, against accumulation of plaque where patients are unable to render effective hygiene in certain parts of the oral cavity. Clinical examples of these applications will be given at the end of the article.

HISTORICAL PERSPECTIVE

There is a spectrum of tooth-colored restorative materials, spanning from GIC at one end to the resin-based materials at the other end. Wilson and McLean introduced the GIC family of materials to the dental profession in 1988.[1] The four families of acid–base materials used in dentistry are: silicate, zinc phosphate, polycarboxylate, and glass-ionomer. They all utilize acid and base components (**Table 1**). It was over 100 years ago when silicate cements were introduced to dentistry as a restorative material. There was anecdotal evidence that silicate cements were an effective anticaries agent that was attributed mainly to the high level of fluoride release from the silicate material. The material's solubility was high, however, and the search for its replacement led to the development of polycarboxylate cements, and eventually GIC. Currently, glass-ionomer is the only restorative material that is water-based and like silicate has an anti-caries effect.[2–4] Current esthetic high-strength GICs are considered to be durable restorative dental cements.[5]

HOW DO GIC ACQUIRE THEIR ANTICARIES EFFECT?

GICs are true acid–base cements where the base is the fluoroaluminosilicate glass powder and the liquid containing acid comes from the polyalkenoic family. In some glass formulations, the F rich phase of the glass can be visible (**Fig. 1**) and physically distinct. Apart from the base and acid, the third major component is water, the major component of the liquid. The total water content of the set cement is somewhere between 11% and 24%. Being a true water-based material, GIC also is recognized as the only biological active restorative material that is currently available.[6]

The precise glass composition varies from one material to another. Traditionally, GIC powder was based on calcium (Ca); however, there are several materials where the calcium has been substituted by strontium (Sr). This was done to impart radiopacity to the material. It is interesting to note that because of their similarity in polarity and atomic size, these two elements are interchangeable in the composition of GIC as well as hydroxyapatite (HAP). Some of the Ca in HAP can be substituted with Sr without any significant disadvantage.[7] It is interesting to note that, at a population level, there is some evidence to show that Sr has anticariogenic properties. Curzon reported on the caries-reducing effect of drinking water containing strontium. He noted a reduction

Table 1		
The acid and base components used in the various dental cements		
Acid-Base Cement	**Acid**	**Base**
Silicate	Calcium-fluoro-alumino-silicate	Phosphoric acid
Zinc Phosphate	Zinc oxide	Phosphoric acid
Polycarboxylate	Zinc oxide	Polyalkenoic acid
Glass-Ionomer	Calcium-fluoro-alumino-silicate	Polyalkenoic acid

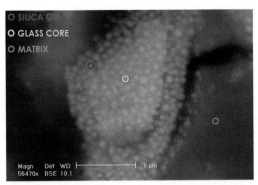

O SILICA GEL
O GLASS CORE
O MATRIX

Magn   Det WD
56470x BSE 10.1   1 µm

Fig. 1. Scanning electron microscope view of a set GIC showing a reacted glass particle in a set cement. The three areas of interest are: the silica ion–depleted gel phase, the glass core with its fluoride-rich phase (dense white droplets), and the matrix of the cement. The minor crack is an artifact.

in DMFT in a population exposed to drinking water containing strontium.[8] The importance of this information will become apparent in the discussion of a study relating to the internal remineralization technique, where both F and Sr from GIC were found to migrate from GIC to the soften dentine left at the base of cavities.

For restorative GIC, approximately 60% of the liquid is water, which plays an important role in the setting reaction and in the final structure of the set cement, as well as contributing to the observed biocompatibility and the well known ionic exchange. Water allows the acid–base reaction to occur and the migration of the various ions out of and into the matrix of the set cement. When the powder is brought into contact with the liquid, the acidity allows the matrix-forming cations, Ca or Sr and Al, to leach out of the glass. These will cross-link with the polyalkenoic chains to form metal polyacrylate salts, which form the matrix and solidify the mix.[9]

MOISTURE CONTROL AND THE CLINICAL PERFORMANCE OF GIC

The setting reaction of GIC is a two-phase process.[6,10] In the first phase, immediately after mixing, there is cross-linking of the poly-acid chains by either the Ca or Sr ions. This cross-linking during this first phase is not stable and can be easily affected by excessive water loss or gain. Clinically, this means that the restoration must be protected, against initial water contamination and desiccation, immediately after placement. In the second phase, within the solidified cement, the poly-acid chains are further cross-linked by trivalent Al ions. This second phase gives the material increased physical properties and reduced solubility.

In the set GIC, water molecules can be classified as either loosely bound or tightly bound. As the material matures, the ratio between the loosely bound and tightly bound water decreases, and the material will show increased in physical properties. This is important for two reasons. First, the loosely bound water is essential for ion release and uptake, and second, it is important to maintain the water balance right through the life of a GIC restoration. Early exposure to excess water during setting and desiccation, at any stage, will lead to poor clinical performance.

ION EXCHANGE BETWEEN GIC AND THE EXTERNAL ENVIRONMENT

Because of the combined effect of release and uptake of ions, GIC is a rich reservoir of apatite forming ions such as fluoride, calcium, strontium, and phosphate. In the aqueous environment of the oral cavity, these are released through an ion exchange process with the environment. There is a natural exchange between Sr and Ca ions.[11] As Sr leaves the set cement, an equivalent number of Ca ions from saliva enter the matrix of the cement to maintain electrolytic balance (**Fig. 2**). Nicholson postulated that this leads to the hardening of the surface, and this was confirmed by Okada when it was found that the surface hardness of a GIC can increase by 39% after 40 days storage in natural saliva.[11–13] This was demonstrated by immersing 24 hours-old buttons of strontium containing GICs in an artificial saliva solution, and then a distribution map of Ca was acquired using electron probe micro analysis (EPMA), which clearly showed that Ca was exchanged for Sr in the matrix of the surface layer of the GIC buttons (see **Fig. 2**). It was postulated that the increase in surface hardness was related to the exchange of Sr by Ca in the matrix; however, the mechanism involved has not yet been identified. This phenomenon means that an exposure to Ca-rich saliva is beneficial to the long-term clinical performance of GIC.

One of the major advantages of GIC is the long-term release of fluoride and other ions. This is characterized by an initial high peak that will decline rapidly to a lower level and sustained over a number of years.[14] It has been shown that there is a topping-up effect[15,16] with the material up-taking fluoride from external sources such as toothpaste and topical fluoride gel. Wilson studied this over a period of 20 months and found that these species still were being released at the end of the experimental period, although at a diminished rate.[17] This fluoride release also can suppress the acidogenicity of the biofilm.[18] From the above observations and what is known about the importance of fluoride in the demineralization and remineralization process, one can understand the protective effect that GIC has on tooth structure in its immediate

Fig. 2. An elemental distribution map showing Ca (*purple*) in the matrix of a Sr-based GIC that was stored in saliva for 7 days.

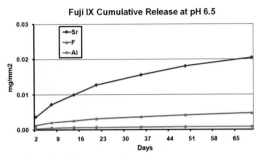

Fig. 3. Cumulative release of Sr, F, and Al into solution.

vicinity.[2] As the level of fluoride, and other ions, in GIC can be recharged, this class of material can be used as a reservoir for fluoride and may act as a slow F release device. GIC also can provide protection by the combined effect of mechanical and chemical means. For example, GIC can be used successfully to protect fissures, and despite a lower retention rate than resin-based fissure sealants, there is evidence that it reduces caries incidence in permanent teeth.[19] In addition, a long-term clinical trial reported an effective rate of 80.6%, and suggested traditional retention is not essential for caries prevention.[20] This is probably due to the effect of the chemical protection the material provides, and the fact that GIC tends to fail cohesively, so there is always a remaining layer on the surface, even when GIC is no longer clinically detectable.

This ion exchange is not only restricted to fluoride. The essential elements in a GIC include Ca, or Sr, Al, Si, and F. After the completion of the setting reaction, a portion of these ions is available for transfer from the matrix to the surrounding environment. As shown in (**Fig. 3**), the level of release of Sr far exceeds that of F or Al ions. It is well accepted that the release is caused by an exchange process, so it is unlikely to adversely affect the clinical performance of the material.

The following segment looks at some new clinical indications where the biocompatibility effect of GIC is important for clinical success.

ION EXCHANGE BETWEEN GIC AND CARIOUS DENTINE

The term internal remineralization was introduced to describe the interaction between GIC and carious dentine, and to suggest that GIC is an essential tool in the

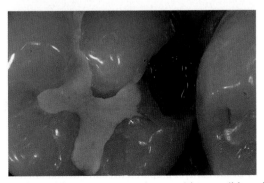

Fig. 4. Initial presentation with symptoms consistent with reversible pulpitis.

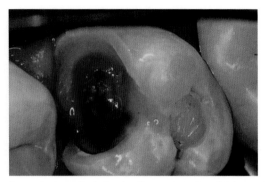

Fig. 9. The gingival margin is entirely in dentine; a margin of 2-mm wide was created in sound dentine and the soft dentine, over the pulpal wall, was removed by hand and conditioned using 10% polyalkenoic acid.

When GIC is placed in direct contact with affected dentine, the migration of apatite-forming elements F and Sr from the GIC to carious dentine can be extensive. In a clinical trial study,[3] these two elements were found to have accumulated deep into the lesion with the maximum depth reaching over 1.5 mm. The controlling factor was the depth of the lesion and the physical state of the demineralized dentine.

The clinical application of the internal remineralization concept is illustrated in the following clinical case. A patient presented with a proximal cavity and reported mild symptoms consistent with reversible pulpitis. There was no evidence of periapical involvement. The initial presentation can be seen in **Fig. 4**, with only enough enamel removed to gain proper access to the cavity (**Fig. 5**). Note that the entire enamel margin and dentino-enamel junction have been cleaned to leave 2 mm of sound hard dentine to ensure a seal can be achieved and maintained long-term (**Fig. 6**). Only hand instrumentation was then used in the removal of the soft dentine immediately above the pulp to minimize the risk of direct pulp exposure. The cavity was then conditioned using 10% polyacrylic acid for 10 seconds. Following conditioning, a small amount of high fluoride-releasing GIC was applied over the soft dentine as a liner. The cavity then was restored with composite resin in the conventional manner. The selection of composite resin for the final restoration was based on the fact that there was sufficient enamel still available right around the periphery of the cavity (see **Fig. 6**).

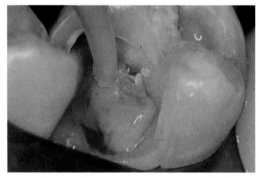

Fig. 10. A high fluoride-releasing GIC liner is applied to the discolored portion for internal remineralization.

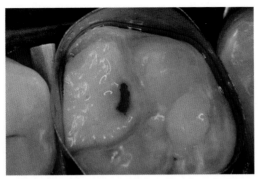

Fig. 11. A base of high-strength GIC is placed to ensure a long-lasting seal along the dentine margin.

It is suggested that GIC, through its self-adhesive characteristics, will provide a complete and long-lasting seal, preventing the ingress of bacteria and potential nutrients. GIC can be placed in close proximity to the pulp without the risk of inducing irreversible inflammation and the placement of calcium hydroxide is no longer needed, unless there is a direct pulp exposure. Providing that the restoration is completely sealed then there is no risk in leaving the demineralized dentin under the GIC lining.

THE SANDWICH TECHNIQUE

This technique uses two different materials for the final restoration, and some clinicians use the following analogy to describe the rationale for its use; GIC is used as a dentine replacement, while composite resin acts as an enamel replacement. The indication is badly broken down teeth or when part of the gingival margin is located on dentine, because there is doubt on the long-term performance of a dentin adhesive in the absence of enamel.[26] The following clinical case is an example of combining the internal remineralization, to treat carious dentine, and sandwich techniques, to restore the tooth. This patient presented with a large proximal lesion and reported mild symptoms over a brief period (**Figs. 7** and **8**). A clean margin of 2 mm wide was created using a round bur, and only hand instruments were used to remove carious dentine. The finished cavity was treated with 10% polyacrylic acid for 10 seconds. Note that the enamel transverse ridge was retained so not to weaken the tooth crown (**Fig. 9**).

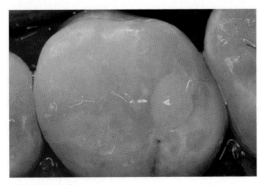

Fig. 12. Final sandwich restoration.

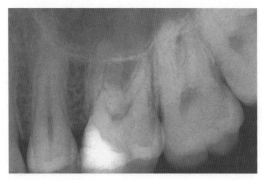

Fig. 13. Radiograph of final restoration.

The discolored dentine was treated with a high F-releasing GIC liner (**Fig. 10**). A high-strength GIC was laid down as a base in preparation for the composite resin restoration. This was done to ensure a long-lasting seal along the gingival margin (**Figs. 11–13**), The three practical advantages of this technique are that it

- Minimizes the risk of pulp exposure
- Minimizes the number of increments of composite resin to be placed, offering time savings
- Results in a longlasting seal around the dentine margin.

SURFACE PROTECTION FOR ROOT SURFACES IN ELDERLY PATIENTS

One of the new challenges clinicians are facing is the maintenance of good oral health in the older patients. Reinhardt predicted that by the year 2030 the number of retained teeth in people living in the United States, aged between 45 to 84, will be approximately 2.2 billion compared with just over 1 billion in 1990. He recognized these teeth will exist in a more hostile oral environment.

Root caries can be defined as caries lesions initiated on exposed root surfaces. At an early stage, they are difficult to detect visually, because the first changes are in surface hardness and texture of the affected areas. Unlike enamel lesions, discoloration comes much later, and they are usually masked by plaque and inflammation of the surrounding soft tissue. Once established, the lesions can spread incisally by

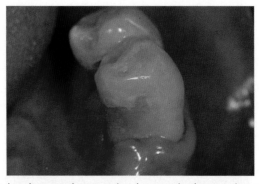

Fig. 14. An exposed and arrested root caries that required protection as the patient could no longer maintain good oral hygiene because of arthritis.

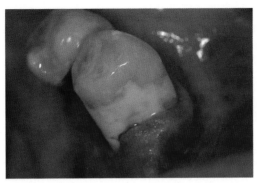

Fig. 15. The root surface is now protected with a thin film of GIC.

undermining the thin enamel at the CEJ, but more often, they spread below the gum level. These lesions quickly become cavitated, because dentin contains much less mineral than enamel, and more is permeable because of the presence of dentinal tubules. In the following clinical case, GIC was applied as a therapeutic coating to protect the exposed root surfaces and lesions. The original caries lesion had been arrested for many years (**Fig. 14**). This had been achieved with a combination of good oral hygiene, use of a high fluoride-containing toothpaste, and daily application of a calcium and phosphate-containing paste to saturate the biofilm. The lesion displayed the three characteristics of a remineralized dentine surface; it was discolored, shiny, and hard. However, with the onset of arthritis, the task of keeping the area clean became too much of a challenge for the patient. After a period of assessment, it was decided that the area should be protected with a thin coat of high fluoride-releasing GIC, Fuji Triage (Fuji VII, GC Corp, Tokyo, Japan) (**Fig. 15**). Being a conventional GIC, this thin film GIC adheres well to the root surface and acts as a mechanical barrier to protect the area and minimize plaque accumulation. It releases significantly much more F than the traditional restorative GICs and if recharged with a daily exposure to fluoridated toothpaste, then the F release can be maintained indefinitely. A thin film of half a millimeter or less will allow ions such as calcium and fluoride to cross from saliva to the underlying root surface and remineralize it further.

SUMMARY

GIC is an important tool in the fight against dental caries, and it should be used in conjunction with other traditional tools:

- It can be thought of as a reservoir of fluoride and other ions in the oral cavity. Externally it can be used as a therapeutic coating to protect the tooth surface against acid and to modulate bacterial activities.
- It assists in preserving carious dentine at the base of restoration, by delivering F and other apatite-forming ions, and providing a long-lasting seal to both dentine and enamel.
- GIC can be used as a restorative material, a liner, a base, a luting cement, a fissure sealant, and a surface protectant.

The dental profession has come to the realization that to control caries effectively, it is necessary to move from the surgical-only approach to a combined surgical–medical approach with special focus on engaging patients in changing their lifestyle. GIC, as a family of materials, is part of the armamentarium that the clinician has for the management of dental caries, as it can contribute to the surgical and medical management components.

REFERENCES

1. Wilson AD, McLean JW. Glass-ionomer cement. London: Quintessence; 1988.
2. ten Cate JM, van Duinen RN. Hypermineralization of dentinal lesions adjacent to glass-ionomer cement restorations. J Dent Res 1995;74(6):1266–71.
3. Ngo HC, Mount G, McIntyre J, et al. Chemical exchange between glass-ionomer restorations and residual carious dentine in permanent molars: an in vivo study. J Dent 2006;34(8):608–13.
4. Smales RJ, Ngo HC, Yip KH, et al. Clinical effects of glass ionomer restorations on residual carious dentin in primary molars. Am J Dent 2005;18(3):188–93.
5. Mount GJ. Glass ionomers: a review of their current status. Oper Dent 1999;24(2): 115–24.
6. Mount G. An atlas of glass-ionomer cements. A clinician's guide. London: Martin Dunitz; 2002.
7. Featherstone JD, Shields CP, Khademazad B, et al. Acid reactivity of carbonated apatites with strontium and fluoride substitutions. J Dent Res 1983;62:1049–53.
8. Curzon ME, Adkins BL. Combined effect of trace elements and fluorine on caries. J Dent Res 1970;49:526–9.
9. Wilson AD, Crisp S, Ferner AJ. Reactions in Glass-ionomer Cements: IV. Effect of chelating comonomers on setting behaviour. J Dent 1974;55(3):489–95.
10. Wilson AD. Secondary reactions in glass-ionomer cements. J Mater Sci Lett 1996; 15:275–6.
11. Ngo H, Marino V, Mount GJ. Calcium, strontium, aluminium, sodium, and fluoride release from four glass ionomer cements. J Dent 1998;77:75.
12. Nicholson JW. Chemistry of glass-ionomer cements: a review. Biomaterials 1998; 19:485–94.
13. Okada K, Tosaki S, Hirota K, et al. Surface hardness change of restorative filling materials stored in saliva. Dent Mater 2001;17(1):34–9.
14. Forsten L. Fluoride release and uptake by glass-ionomers and related materials and its clinical effect. Biomaterials 1998;19:503–8.
15. Forsten L. Fluoride release of glass-ionomers. Presented at the 2nd Symposium on Glass Ionomers. Philadelphia, 1994.
16. Cranfield M, Kuhn AT, Winter G. Factors relating to the rates of fluoride release from a glass-ionomer cement. J Dent 1982;10:333–4.
17. Wilson AD, Groffman DM, Kuhn AT. The release of fluoride and other chemical species from a glass-ionomer cement. Biomaterials 1985;6(6):431–3.
18. Hengtrakool C, Pearson GJ, Wilson M. Interaction between GIC and S sanguis biofilms: antibacterial properties and changes of surface hardness. J Dent 2006;34(8):588–97.
19. Beauchamp J, Caufield PW, Crall JP, et al. Evidence-based clinical recommendations for the use of pit-and-fissure sealants: a report of the American Dental Association Council on Scientific Affairs. J Am Dent Assoc 2008;139(3):257–68.
20. Arrow P, Riordan PJ. Retention and caries preventive effects of a GIC and a resin-based fissure sealant. Community Dent Oral Epidemiol 1995;23(5):282–5.
21. Fusayama T, Okuse K, Hosoda J. Relationship between hardness, discoloration, and microbial invasion in carious dentin. J Dent Res 1966;45(4):1033–46.

22. Massler M. Changing concepts in the treatment of carious lesions. Br Dent J 1967;123(11):547–8.
23. Mertz-Fairhurst EJ, Smith CD, Williams JE, et al. Cariostatic and ultraconservative sealed restorations: six-year results. Quintessence Int 1992;23(12):827–38.
24. Mertz Fairhurst EJ, Curtis JW, Ergle JW, et al. Ultraconservative and cariostatic sealed restorations: results at year 10. J Am Dent Assoc 1998;129:55–66.
25. Kidd EA. How 'clean' must a cavity be before restoration? Caries Res 2004;38(3): 305–13.
26. De Munck J, Van Meerbeek B, Yoshida Y, et al. Four-year water degradation of total-etch adhesives bonded to dentin. J Dent Res 2003;82(2):136–40.

Assessment and Management of Dental Erosion

Xiaojie Wang, DMD, PhD*, Adrian Lussi, Ms of Chem DMD, PhD

KEYWORDS

• Tooth erosion • Risk factors • Diagnosis • Prevention

The pattern of oral disease has been influenced by the ever-changing human lifestyle. Tooth wear, especially tooth erosion, has drawn increasing attention as a risk factor for tooth damage or loss. Dental erosion and caries lesions result from acids on tooth structure. The acids causing caries lesions are produced by bacteria in the mouth. The acids that are responsible for tooth erosion, on the other hand, stem from extrinsic (eg, soft drinks, acidic foods) or intrinsic (eg, reflux fluid) sources. Structurally, caries lesions are characterized by a subsurface partial demineralization in which the subsurface lesion body is covered by an intact surface layer (**Fig. 1**, *left*). By comparison, tooth erosion is characterized by initial surface softening and subsequent bulk material loss. In the early stage, acids diffuse into the tooth and remove calcium and phosphate ions from the outer few micrometers of hard tissues, forming a demineralized, weakened overlying layer. In the advanced stage, the apatite crystals of the tooth are destroyed and dissolved away layer by layer from the tooth surface, leading to a generalized loss of tooth volume (**Fig. 1**, *right*).

There is some evidence that the prevalence of dental erosion is growing.[1] In a study in the United Kingdom, 1308 adolescents of mixed ethnicities were examined at the age of 12 years and then 2 years later. Almost 5% of the subjects at baseline and more than 13% 2 years later had deep enamel or dentin lesions. In this study, approximately 12% of the erosion-free adolescents developed erosive lesions in the following 2 years.[2] The spread of tooth erosion, especially in children, adolescents, and young adults, has been largely linked to the high consumption of acidic drinks and foods. However, it is impossible to avoid potentially erosive agents from contact with the teeth during a lifetime. After applying rehabilitation treatment, restorative materials also exhibit degradation in acids. Therefore, to prevent or inhibit further erosion, the emphasis should be on early diagnosis and adequate preventive strategies. Restorative measures should be taken only when tooth loss caused by erosive wear reaches a certain threshold.

Department of Preventive, Restorative and Pediatric Dentistry, School of Dental Medicine, University of Bern, Freiburgstrasse 7, CH - 3010 Bern, Switzerland
* Corresponding author.
E-mail address: xiaojie.wang@zmk.unibe.ch

Dent Clin N Am 54 (2010) 565–578
doi:10.1016/j.cden.2010.03.003
0011-8532/10/$ – see front matter © 2010 Elsevier Inc. All rights reserved.

dental.theclinics.com

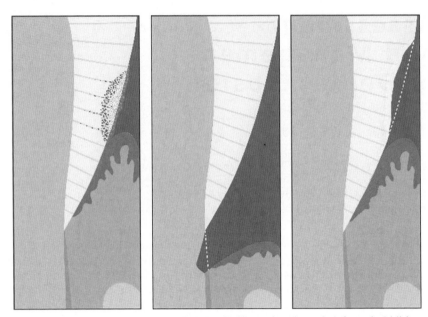

Fig. 1. Comparison of the pattern of caries (*left*), wedge-shaped defects (*middle*), and erosion with the intact enamel adjacent to the gingiva (*right*).

DIAGNOSIS

In the early stages, it is difficult to diagnose erosion, as erosion is associated with few signs and fewer, if any, symptoms such as pain or sensitivity. There is no device available in routine dental practice for the specific detection of dental erosion and its progression. Therefore, clinical appearance has to be applied as the most important feature for dental professionals to diagnose tooth erosion.[3] In the more advanced stages, dentin may become exposed. To determine this condition, disclosing agents can be used to render dentin visible.

The appearance of smooth, silky-glazed, sometimes dull enamel with the absence of perikymata and intact enamel along the gingival margin are some typical signs of enamel erosion. An enamel ridge may persist at the crown margin. The presence of this phenomenon can be explained on the one hand by plaque residues, which can act as a diffusion barrier to acids, and on the other hand by sulcular fluid, which leads to neutralization of the acids in the gingival region.[4] The initial features of erosion on occlusal and incisal surfaces are the same as described earlier. Further progression of occlusal erosion leads to a rounding of the cusps and restorations rising above the level of the adjacent tooth surfaces. In severe cases, the entire occlusal morphology disappears. Extensive loss of enamel can lead to dentin exposure and even lead to pulp exposure in some extreme cases.[5] The exposed surface becomes sensitive to cold and warm foods and to tactile stimuli. To record the progress of the erosion, photographs or models should be taken periodically. **Fig. 2** shows the typical pattern of dental erosions.

Erosion has to be distinguished from attrition and abrasion. For the latter, tooth surfaces are often flat, with glossy areas with distinct margins and corresponding features on the antagonistic teeth. It is not always possible to differentiate these wear lesions because they frequently occur simultaneously with different proportional

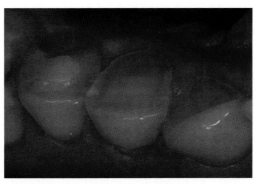

Fig. 2. Occlusal erosive tooth wear with involvement of dentin. The composite filling rises above the level of the adjacent tooth surface, a clear sign of an erosive process. Decalcification can be seen in the proximal area of the first premolar.

effects.[6] As the tooth enamel layer demineralizes and becomes softened it becomes more susceptible to abrasion and attrition. Facial erosion should be distinguished from wedge-shaped defects, which are located at, or apical to, the enamel-cementum junction, as shown in **Fig. 3**. The coronal part of wedge-shaped defects ideally has a sharp margin and cuts at a right angle into the enamel surface, whereas the apical part bottoms out to the root surface. Thereby the depth of the defect exceeds its width. In addition, tooth surfaces of patients with active (unstained) erosion often have no caries lesions. However, caries lesions may occur in patients with erosion at sites where plaque accumulation is possible (eg, approximal; see **Fig. 2**).

The Basic Erosive Wear Examination (BEWE) was introduced to facilitate quantifying the risk of erosion.[7] It can be used with the diagnostic criteria of most current indices and allows reanalysis and integration of results from existing studies. All teeth, except third molars, are examined in each case from the vestibular, occlusal, and palatial aspects for acid damage. The most severely affected surface in a sextant is recorded with a 4-level score (**Table 1**). The sum of the scores defines the severity of erosive wear and guides the further management of the condition (**Table 2**). The maximum score per subject is 18. Management includes identification and elimination of the main causative factor(s), prevention, and monitoring, as well as symptomatic and operative intervention, where appropriate.

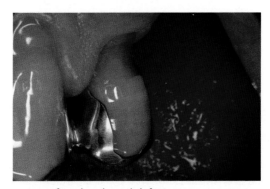

Fig. 3. Clinical appearance of wedge-shaped defects.

Table 1
Criteria for grading erosive wear

Score	Criteria
0	No erosive tooth wear
1	Initial loss of surface texture
2[a]	Distinct defect, hard tissue loss <50% of the surface area
3[a]	Hard tissue loss ≥50% of the surface area

[a] With scores 2 and 3, dentin is often involved.

From Bartlett D, Ganss C, Lussi A. Basic Erosive Wear Examination (BEWE): a new scoring system for scientific and clinical needs. Clin Oral Investig 2008;12 (Suppl 1):S65–8.

RISK FACTORS

Tooth erosion is a multifactorial condition and has a complex etiology. Various factors involved in the generation and development of erosion may be patient dependent or nutrition dependent (**Fig. 4**).[8,9] Every factor plays a more or less important role in inducing or preventing erosion. With time, the interaction of all factors with the tooth surface may either wear tooth hard tissues away or indeed protect them, depending on their fine balance.

Nutritional Factors

Excessive consumption of acidic foods and drinks is regarded as an important factor leading to tooth erosion. In recent years, the total amount and frequency of consumption of acidic foods and drinks has increased as a result of changes in lifestyles. In 2007, the worldwide annual consumption of soft drinks reached 552 billion liters, the equivalent of just less than 83 L per person per year, and this is projected to

Table 2
Complexity levels as a guide to clinical management

Susceptibility Level	Cumulative Score of All Sextants	Management
	≤2	Routine maintenance and observation Repeat at 3-year intervals
Low	3–8	Oral hygiene and dietary assessment and advice. Identify the main causative factor(s) and develop strategies to eliminate their effects, routine maintenance, and observation. Repeat at 1- to 2-year intervals
Medium	9–13	As above plus Measures to increase the resistance of tooth surfaces Ideally, avoid the placement of restorations and monitor erosive wear with study casts, photographs, or silicone impressions Repeat at 6- to 12-month intervals
High	≥14	As above plus Especially in cases of severe progression consider special care, which may involve restorations Repeat at 6-month intervals

From Bartlett D, Ganss C, Lussi A. Basic Erosive Wear Examination (BEWE): a new scoring system for scientific and clinical needs. Clin Oral Investig 2008;12 (Suppl 1):S65–8.

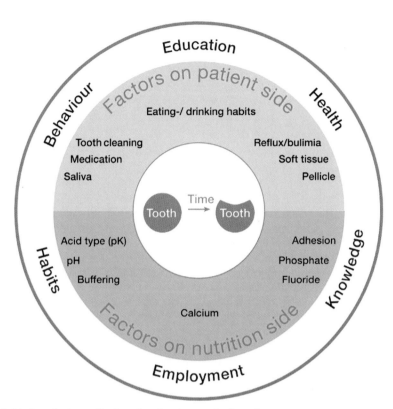

Fig. 4. Various factors affecting the development of erosion.

increase to 95 L per person per year by 2012. However, the figure has already reached an average of 212 L per person per year in the United States in 2009.[10] The erosion potential of a drink or food is codetermined by its chemical and physical properties, such as the pH value, the levels of calcium, phosphate, and to a lesser extent fluoride, and the titratable acidity (buffering capacity), as well as the adhesiveness and displacement of the potentially erosive substances.

The pH value is an important but not the only variable in the erosive potential of drinks and foods. Apart from its pH value, the ability of an acidic solution to dissolve enamel or dentin depends on its ability to keep pH unaffected by the dissolution of tooth mineral and dilution with saliva (ie, its buffering capacity).[11] Buffering capacity is associated with the undissociated acid in drinks and foods. Undissociated acid is not charged and can diffuse into the hard tissues of the teeth and act as a buffer to maintain the H^+ concentration. Consequently, the driving force for demineralization at the site of dissolution is maintained.[12,13] This parameter, therefore, may be a good indicator of the erosive potential of a food or drink, especially after exposure for a certain time.[14,15] The greater the buffering capacity of the drink, the longer it will take for saliva to neutralize the acid and then the more apatite may be dissolved before an higher pH value is reached and dissolution ceases.

The concentration of calcium (Ca), phosphate (P), and fluoride (F) ions in a drink or food also plays a key role in tooth erosion. Combined with the pH value, they determine the degree of saturation with respect to enamel or dentin, which is the driving force for dissolution. Solutions supersaturated with respect to enamel or dentin will not dissolve it. A low degree of undersaturation leads to an initial surface demineralization, which is followed by a local increase in pH and increased mineral ions content in the liquid surface layer adjacent to the tooth surface. This layer then becomes saturated with respect to tooth mineral and does not demineralize the tooth further. Yoghurt is a good example of a food with low pH value (pH ~4) leading to no erosion. This fact can be attributed to its supersaturation with respect to tooth mineral resulting from the high Ca and P concentration. Modified diets with minerals (eg, Ca, P, or casein phosphopeptide-amorphous calcium phosphate [CPP-ACP]), showed a reduced erosive capacity and therefore were recommended to patients at risk of erosion.[16–19] However, the addition of minerals to the diet may only retard enamel dissolution, rather than completely prevent its progression.

Common extrinsic dietary acids include citric acid, phosphoric acid, ascorbic acid, malic acid, and carbonic acid. Citric acid is known to exhibit a greater erosive potential than the others. The greater erosive potential of citric acid might be related to its ability to form chelating complexes with Ca and/or high buffering capacity. A study by Meurman and ten Cate (1996) showed that up to 32% of the Ca in saliva could be complexed by citrate at concentrations common in fruit juices, thus reducing the supersaturation of saliva and increasing the driving force for dissolution with respect to tooth mineral.[20] Therefore, acids such as citric acid have a twofold effect and may be very damaging to the tooth surface.[21] The erosive potential of acidic dietary substances may be decreased by replacing highly erosive acids (eg, citric acid) with acids with lower erosive potential.

The adhesiveness and displacement of the liquid are other factors to be considered in the erosive process. There seem to be differences in the ability of beverages to adhere to enamel based on their thermodynamic properties.[22] However, further research is needed to understand this phenomenon better.

Patient Factors

In tooth erosion, risk factors such as lifestyle, oral hygiene habits, and health condition are patient modifiable.

The manner in which dietary acids are introduced into the mouth (sipping, sucking, with/without drinking straw), which determines the duration and the localization of the acid attack, influences the appearance of the erosions.[23–25] The frequency and duration of acid attacks are also closely associated with erosion and, therefore, very important for the adoption of prophylactic measures.[26–29] Contact of the teeth with acids during the night can also lead to erosion because of the reduced production of saliva. Thus, for example, apart from cariogenesis there can be massive erosive tooth structure destruction as a result of the consumption of acidic sweet drinks, which some infants drink from their bottles continuously during the night.

Another risk factor on the patient side is stomach acid, which enters the mouth as a consequence of vomiting or reflux. Vomiting is the forceful expulsion of the contents of one's stomach through the mouth and sometimes the nose. This phenomenon normally results from psychological disorders such as anorexia and bulimia nervosa. Reflux is defined as the involuntary movement of the gastric contents from the stomach into the mouth, caused by some abnormality in the gastrointestinal tract. In general, acidic gastric content entering the mouth may, in time, erode the teeth. Unlike dietary acids, the pH and titratability of gastric juice is significantly greater and so the level of destruction is normally more severe.[30] Because the clinical manifestation of dental erosion does not occur until gastric acid has acted on the dental hard tissues regularly over some time, dental erosion caused by gastric acid has been observed only in those diseases that are associated with chronic vomiting or persistent gastroesophageal reflux, also known as gastroesphageal reflux disease (GERD), over a long period. Intrinsic tooth erosion usually takes place in the region of the occlusal and palatal tooth surfaces of the maxillary teeth. Often the dentist is the first person to detect these diseases and should treat them accordingly.

Saliva is of the essence in the tooth erosion process. Several salivary protective mechanisms come into play during an erosive challenge: dilution and clearance of an erosive agent from the mouth, neutralization and buffering of acids, slowing down the rate of enamel dissolution through the common ion effect by salivary Ca and P, and involvement in the formation of the pellicle.[31] The acquired pellicle is an organic film free of bacteria that covers oral hard and soft tissues. It is composed of mucins, glycoproteins and proteins, including several enzymes.[32] The acquired pellicle may protect against erosion by acting as a diffusion barrier or a selectively permeable membrane preventing direct contact between the acids and the tooth surface, thus reducing the dissolution rate of dental hard tissues.

Practical experience demonstrates the importance of saliva in patients suffering from salivary flow impairment. Studies have shown that erosion may be associated with low salivary flow or low buffering capacity.[26,29,33] The dry mouth condition is usually related to aging,[34–36] even though some other studies have not identified this correlation.[37,38] It is well established that patients taking medication can also present decreased salivary output,[39] as well as those who have received radiation therapy for head and neck cancer.[40] Tests of the stimulated and unstimulated flow rate, as well as the buffering capacity of saliva may provide some information about the susceptibility of an individual to dental erosion. However, these parameters are only 2 aspects of a multifactorial condition. Sialometric evaluations should be performed at a fixed time point or in a limited time interval in the morning, to avoid intra-individual variation as a result of the circadian cycle. Studies have shown that sour foodstuffs have strong influences on the anticipatory salivary flow,[41,42] which can be significantly increased compared with the normal unstimulated flow rate.[43] Hypersalivation also occurs in advance of vomiting as a response from the vomiting center of the brain,[44] as frequently seen in individuals suffering from anorexia and bulimia nervosa, rumination, or chronic alcoholism. It is suggested that this could minimize the erosion caused by acids of gastric origin. On the other hand, patients with symptoms of GERD should not expect salivary output to increase before gastric juice reflux, because this is an involuntary response that is not coordinated by the autonomic nervous system.[45] Therefore, there may be insufficient time for saliva to act before erosion occurs.

Millward and colleagues[23] monitored the pH at the surface of teeth in healthy volunteers after drinking 1% citric acid. They observed that the pH recovered to more than pH 5.5 within 2 minutes at a site adjacent to the palatal surface of the upper central incisor and within 4 to 5 minutes at another palatal surface on the upper first molar. Thus, the clearance rate of erosive agents may be influenced by the anatomy of the teeth and soft tissues, by the movement of the tongue and buccal mucosa, as well as by the swallowing pattern. In addition, the mechanical abrasion caused by the tongue was considered to be a contributing factor in erosion.[46,47]

Apart from the risk factors discussed earlier, occupation and sport may also lead to erosive wear. Employees in the chemical industry or professional wine tasters have a higher risk of suffering erosion as a result of the increased acid-tooth contact.[48,49] Tooth erosion associated with professional athletes or excessive exercise has also been reported.[50] Excessive exposure to water or sports drinks with low pH, or increased gastroesophageal reflux resulting from strenuous exercise may be responsible for the sport-induced erosion.[50] In the occurrence and development of erosion, occupation and sport can only be considered as cofactors rather than isolated factors, because erosion is a multifactorial condition.

PREVENTIVE MEASURES

Tooth erosion is an irreversible process and may eventually require extensive and expensive prosthetic measures. Preventive strategies, therefore, play a vital role in decreasing erosive wear and maintaining the safety and efficacy of restorative treatment as long as possible. Dental professionals must have a strong understanding of the causative factors for erosion when they start an individually targeted preventive strategy. The goal of preventive strategies is to reduce the exposure of the teeth to extrinsic and/or intrinsic acids and to enhance the preventive capability of the teeth against erosion (**Table 3**).

When dietary acids are deemed to be the main causative factor, prophylaxis focuses primarily on reducing acid exposure. Diet modification is not patient dependent and should be recommended. The consumption of potentially harmful drinks and foods should be limited to main meals only. Finishing eating or drinking with dairy

Table 3 Recommendations for patients at high risk for dental erosion	
Control of the acid action	Reduce acid exposure by reducing the frequency and contact time of acids (main meals only)
	Do not hold or swish acidic drinks in your mouth. Avoid sipping these drinks. Drink cold drinks that are less erosive
	Consider intake of modified food and beverages with no or reduced erosive potential
	After an erosive challenge (vomiting, acidic diet), use a (tin- and) fluoride-containing mouth rinse, a sodium bicarbonate (baking soda) solution, milk, cheese, or sugar-free yoghurt. If none of these is possible, rinse with water
	After acid intake, stimulate saliva flow with chewing gum or lozenges
Control of dental hygiene	Avoid tooth brushing immediately *after* an erosive challenge, instead brush before
	Use a soft toothbrush and low abrasion fluoride-containing toothpaste
	Periodically, gently apply (tin-containing) fluoride mouth rinse. Use concentrated topical fluoride (slightly acidic formulations are preferable, as they form CaF_2 at a higher rate)
Control of endogenous acid exposure	Suspicion of reflux: referral to gastroenterologist
	Anorexia-bulimia patients: arrange for psychological or psychiatric care
	Avoid reflux-inducing foods, eg, citrus products, vinegar, high fat foods (fried foods, high fat dairy products, high fat meats and so forth.), tomato, peppermint, coffee, carbonated beverages, chocolate
	Eat several small meals each day instead of 3 large ones. Avoid a big meal before bedtime
	Use chewing gum to reduce postprandial reflux after eating
	Use acid block: proton pump inhibitors

Modified from Lussi A, Hellwig E, Ganss C, et al. Buonocore memorial lecture. Dental erosion. Oper Dent 2009;34(3):251–62; with permission.

products (eg, milk, cheese, or sugar-free yoghurt) may promote rehardening of softened dental enamel. After meals, other strategies, that stimulate salivary flow (eg, chewing gum) or directly help neutralize acids (eg, rinsing with sodium bicarbonate), may counter the destructive effects of dietary acids.[51,52] Chewing gum after a meal may also help to reduce postprandial esophageal acid exposure[53] and is beneficial to reduce erosion caused by symptomatic reflux.[54,55] Some eating habits, such as sipping, swishing or holding drinks in the mouth, should be avoided because they prolong the acid-tooth contact time and increase the susceptibility of teeth to erosion.

Recent studies have shown that fluoride preparations with polyvalent metal cations, such as tin ion, are potential erosion inhibitors.[56–59] The topical application of fluoride is another strategy for strengthening tooth surfaces against tooth erosion. The protective effect of fluoride could be as a result of the precipitation of CaF_2-like materials on the tooth surface; they are thicker the more concentrated and acidic the preparation is.[60] However, the deposited CaF_2-like layer is inclined to be dissolved in acids. The long-term and frequent application of fluoride-containing products is essential to inhibit tooth erosion.

Oral hygiene measures may influence the progress of erosive lesions. To enhance the resistance of teeth against mechanical challenge, brushing the teeth was recommended after waiting for at least 30 minutes to 1 hour after eating and drinking.[61,62] During this period, the remineralization/rehardening of softened tooth enamel by saliva was expected. However, compared with demineralized but unbrushed teeth, enamel loss for the demineralized and brushed teeth (≤ 1 hour) was still much higher.[63] In an in vitro study by Eisenburger and colleagues,[64] it was suggested that a 6-hour remineralization time should be reached to completely reharden the softened enamel. In this study no salivary proteins were involved, which enhanced remineralization. In a study using human saliva, no significant protection against toothbrush abrasion was found up to 6 hours.[65] Recently, it was suggested that brushing the teeth before an erosive attack is likely to reduce erosive tooth loss. When erosion is a problem, brushing the teeth before an acid attack should be recommended using a soft-bristled toothbrush and a low abrasive toothpaste. This procedure does not completely remove the pellicle. Therefore, the pellicle is able to continue fulfilling some protective function in the following erosive attack.[66]

To eradicate intrinsic tooth erosion, causal systemic therapy must be initiated. Patients with anorexia and bulimia require psychological or psychiatric therapy. For patients with reflux, accurate clarification of the cause with subsequent treatment (general medicine or surgical intervention) should be undertaken.

RESTORATIVE TREATMENT

When substance loss caused by erosive tooth wear reaches a certain level, oral rehabilitation becomes necessary. There are different reasons for restorative treatment: (1) the structural integrity of the tooth is threatened; (2) the exposed dentin is hypersensitive; (3) the erosive defect is esthetically unacceptable to the patient; (4) pulpal exposure is likely to occur. Depending on the degree of tooth wear, restorative treatment can range from placement of bonded composites or glass ionomers in a few isolated areas of tooth erosion, to crowns, dental porcelain veneers, bridges, or even full-mouth reconstruction in cases of severe tooth enamel damage. No matter what strategies are applied, a key principle must be obeyed: selection of the least invasive intervention. Initial restorative treatment should be conservation and use adhesive materials.[67] When teeth wear, the alveolar bone and associated tissues should adapt to the change with alveolar compensation.[68] Despite losing crown height, the intact occlusal relationships cannot supply enough space for the restorative material. To gain interocclusal space with minimal invasion, orthodontic treatment is indicated, especially when groups of teeth (eg, all the teeth in the anterior region) are involved. Orthodontic treatment can be achieved with fixed or removable appliances, such as the Dahl appliance.[68] Following orthodontic treatment, the eroded teeth can then be reconstructed.[69] With the improvements in restorative materials and adhesive techniques, rehabilitation of eroded dentitions may be reached in a less invasive manner.[70] The application of modern, direct restorative materials has the advantage of providing excellent longevity, even in load-bearing situations.[71,72] Recent case reports have shown the successful rehabilitation of eroded dentitions using adhesive techniques.[69,73,74]

Restorative procedures cannot guarantee the desired effectiveness of oral rehabilitation, even if preventive measures are initiated. Several investigations have shown that, under acidic conditions, all dental restorative materials show degradation over time (surface roughness, decrease of surface hardness, substance loss).[75–80] However, ceramic and composite materials seem to exhibit substantial durability.

REFERENCES

1. Lussi A, Jaeggi T. Erosion–diagnosis and risk factors. Clin Oral Investig 2008; 12(Suppl 1):S5–13.
2. Dugmore CR, Rock WP. Awareness of tooth erosion in 12 year old children and primary care dental practitioners. Community Dent Health 2003;20(4):223–7.
3. Lussi A, Hellwig E, Zero D, et al. Erosive tooth wear: diagnosis, risk factors and prevention. Am J Dent 2006;19(6):319–25.
4. Lussi A, Jaeggi T, Zero D. The role of diet in the aetiology of dental erosion. Caries Res 2004;38(Suppl 1):34–44.
5. Gandara BK, Truelove EL. Diagnosis and management of dental erosion. J Contemp Dent Pract 1999;1(1):16–23.
6. Nunn J, Shaw L, Smith A. Tooth wear–dental erosion. Braz Dent J 1996;180(9): 349–52.
7. Bartlett D, Ganss C, Lussi A. Basic Erosive Wear Examination (BEWE): a new scoring system for scientific and clinical needs. Clin Oral Investig 2008; 12(Suppl 1):S65–8.
8. Lussi A, Schaffner M, Jaeggi T, et al. Erosionen. Schweiz Monatsschr Zahnmed 2005;115(10):3–22.
9. Lussi A, Hellwig E. Risk assessment and preventive measures. In: Lussi A, editor. Dental erosion: from diagnosis to therapy. Monographs in oral science. Basel (Switzerland): Karger; 2006. p. 190–9.
10. Packer CD. Cola-induced hypokalaemia: a super-sized problem. Int J Clin Pract 2009;63(6):833–5.
11. Larsen MJ, Nyvad B. Enamel erosion by some soft drinks and orange juices relative to their pH, buffering effect and contents of calcium phosphate. Caries Res 1999;33(1):81–7.
12. Gray JA. Kinetics of the dissolution of human dental enamel in acid. J Dent Res 1962;41(3):633–45.
13. Featherstone JD, Rodgers BE. Effect of acetic, lactic and other organic acids on the formation of artificial carious lesions. Caries Res 1981;15(5):377–85.
14. Owens BM. The potential effects of pH and buffering capacity on dental erosion. Gen Dent 2007;55(6):527–31.

15. Edwards M, Creanor SL, Foye RH, et al. Buffering capacities of soft drinks: the potential influence on dental erosion. J Oral Rehabil 1999;26(12):923–7.
16. Hooper S, West NX, Sharif N, et al. A comparison of enamel erosion by a new sports drink compared to two proprietary products: a controlled, crossover study in situ. J Dent 2004;32(7):541–5.
17. West NX, Hughes JA, Parker DM, et al. Development of low erosive carbonated fruit drinks 2. Evaluation of an experimental carbonated blackcurrant drink compared to a conventional carbonated drink. J Dent 2003;31(5): 361–5.
18. Ramalingam L, Messer LB, Reynolds EC. Adding casein phosphopeptide-amorphous calcium phosphate to sports drinks to eliminate in vitro erosion. Pediatr Dent 2005;27(1):61–7.
19. Panich M, Poolthong S. The effect of casein phosphopeptide-amorphous calcium phosphate and a cola soft drink on in vitro enamel hardness. J Am Dent Assoc 2009;140(4):455–60.
20. Meurman JH, ten Cate JM. Pathogenesis and modifying factors of dental erosion. Eur J Oral Sci 1996;104(2):199–206.
21. Featherstone JDB, Lussi A. Understanding the chemistry of dental erosion. In: Lussi A, editor. Dental erosion: from diagnosis to therapy. Monographs in oral science. Basel (Switzerland): Karger; 2006. p. 66–76.
22. Ireland AJ, McGuinness N, Sherriff M. An investigation into the ability of soft drinks to adhere to enamel. Caries Res 1995;29(6):470–6.
23. Millward A, Shaw L, Harrington E, et al. Continuous monitoring of salivary flow rate and pH at the surface of the dentition following consumption of acidic beverages. Caries Res 1997;31(1):44–9.
24. Edwards M, Ashwood RA, Littlewood SJ, et al. A videofluoroscopic comparison of straw and cup drinking: the potential influence on dental erosion. Braz Dent J 1998;185(5):244–9.
25. Johansson AK, Lingstrom P, Imfeld T, et al. Influence of drinking method on tooth-surface pH in relation to dental erosion. Eur J Oral Sci 2004;112(6): 484–9.
26. Lussi A, Schaffner M. Progression of and risk factors for dental erosion and wedge-shaped defects over a 6-year period. Caries Res 2000;34(2):182–7.
27. O'Sullivan EA, Curzon ME. A comparison of acidic dietary factors in children with and without dental erosion ASDC. J Dent Child 2000;67(3):186–92.
28. Johansson AK, Lingstrom P, Birkhed D. Comparison of factors potentially related to the occurrence of dental erosion in high- and low-erosion groups. Eur J Oral Sci 2002;110(3):204–11.
29. Jarvinen VK, Rytomaa II, Heinonen OP. Risk factors in dental erosion. J Dent Res 1991;70(6):942–7.
30. Bartlett DW, Coward PY. Comparison of the erosive potential of gastric juice and a carbonated drink in vitro. J Oral Rehabil 2001;28(11):1045–7.
31. Zero DT, Lussi A. Etiology of enamel erosion – intrinsic and extrinsic factors. In: Addy M, Embery G, Edgar WM, et al, editors. Tooth wear and sensitivity. London (UK): Martin Dunitz Ltd; 2000. p. 121–39.
32. Hannig C, Hannig M, Attin T. Enzymes in the acquired enamel pellicle. Eur J Oral Sci 2005;113(1):2–13.
33. Rytomaa I, Jarvinen V, Kanerva R, et al. Bulimia and tooth erosion. Acta Odontol Scand 1998;56(1):36–40.
34. Dodds MW, Johnson DA, Yeh CK. Health benefits of saliva: a review. J Dent 2005; 33(3):223–33.

35. Navazesh M, Mulligan RA, Kipnis V, et al. Comparison of whole saliva flow rates and mucin concentrations in healthy Caucasian young and aged adults. J Dent Res 1992;71(6):1275–8.
36. Percival RS, Challacombe SJ, Marsh PD. Flow rates of resting whole and stimulated parotid saliva in relation to age and gender. J Dent Res 1994;73(8):1416–20.
37. Ben-Aryeh H, Shalev A, Szargel R, et al. The salivary flow rate and composition of whole and parotid resting and stimulated saliva in young and old healthy subjects. Biochem Med Metab Biol 1986;36(2):260–5.
38. Heintze U, Birkhed D, Bjorn H. Secretion rate and buffer effect of resting and stimulated whole saliva as a function of age and sex. Swed Dent J 1983;7(6):227–38.
39. Wynn RL, Meiller TF. Drugs and dry mouth. Gen Dent 2001;49(1):10–4.
40. Dreizen S, Brown LR, Daly TE, et al. Prevention of xerostomia-related dental caries in irradiated cancer patients. J Dent Res 1977;56(2):99–104.
41. Christensen CM, Navazesh M. Anticipatory salivary flow to the sight of different foods. Appetite 1984;5(4):307–15.
42. Lee VM, Linden RW. An olfactory-submandibular salivary reflex in humans. Exp Physiol 1992;77(1):221–4.
43. Engelen L, de Wijk RA, Prinz JF, et al. The relation between saliva flow after different stimulations and the perception of flavor and texture attributes in custard desserts. Physiol Behav 2003;78(1):165–9.
44. Lee M, Feldman M. Nausea and vomiting. In: Feldman M, Scharschmidt B, Sleisenger M, editors. Gastrointestinal and liver disease: pathophysiology, diagnosis, management. 6th edition. Philadelphia: Saunders; 1998. p. 117–27.
45. Hara AT, Lussi A, Zero DT. Biological factors. In: Lussi A, editor. Dental erosion: from diagnosis to therapy. Monographs in oral science. Basel (Switzerland): Karger; 2006. p. 88–99.
46. Holst JJ, Lange F. Perimylolysis A contribution towards the genesis of tooth wasting from non-mechanical causes. Acta Odontol Scand 1939;1(1):36–48.
47. Stephan RM. Effects of different types of human foods on dental health in experimental animals. J Dent Res 1966;45(5):1551–61.
48. Wiegand A, Attin T. Occupational dental erosion from exposure to acids: a review. Occup Med (Lond) 2007;57(3):169–76.
49. Chikte UM, Naidoo S, Kolze TJ, et al. Patterns of tooth surface loss among winemakers. SADJ 2005;60(9):370–4.
50. Centerwall BS, Armstrong CW, Funkhouser LS, et al. Erosion of dental enamel among competitive swimmers at a gas-chlorinated swimming pool. Am J Epidemiol 1986;123(4):641–7.
51. Amaechi BT, Higham SM. In vitro remineralisation of eroded enamel lesions by saliva. J Dent 2001;29(5):371–6.
52. Amaechi BT, Higham SM, Edgar WM. Influence of abrasion in clinical manifestation of human dental erosion. J Oral Rehabil 2003;30(4):407–13.
53. Avidan B, Sonnenberg A, Schnell TG, et al. Walking and chewing reduce postprandial acid reflux. Aliment Pharmacol Ther 2001;15(2):151–5.
54. von Schonfeld J, Hector M, Evans DF, et al. Oesophageal acid and salivary secretion: is chewing gum a treatment option for gastro-oesophageal reflux? Digestion 1997;58(2):111–4.
55. Smoak BR, Koufman JA. Effects of gum chewing on pharyngeal and esophageal pH. Ann Otol Rhinol Laryngol 2001;110(12):1117–9.
56. Ganss C, Schlueter N, Hardt M, et al. Effect of fluoride compounds on enamel erosion in vitro: a comparison of amine, sodium and stannous fluoride. Caries Res 2008;42(1):2–7.

57. Schlueter N, Hardt M, Lussi A, et al. Tin-containing fluoride solutions as anti-erosive agents in enamel: an in vitro tin-uptake, tissue-loss, and scanning electron micrograph study. Eur J Oral Sci 2009;117(4):427–34.
58. Schlueter N, Klimek J, Ganss C. Efficacy of an experimental tin-F-containing solution in erosive tissue loss in enamel and dentine in situ. Caries Res 2009; 43(6):415–21.
59. Schlueter N, Klimek J, Ganss C. In vitro efficacy of experimental tin- and fluoride-containing mouth rinses as anti-erosive agents in enamel. J Dent 2009;37(12): 944–8.
60. Saxegaard E, Rolla G. Fluoride acquisition on and in human enamel during topical application in vitro. Scand J Dent Res 1988;96(6):523–35.
61. Jaeggi T, Lussi A. Toothbrush abrasion of erosively altered enamel after intraoral exposure to saliva: an in situ study. Caries Res 1999;33(6):455–61.
62. Wetton S, Hughes J, West N, et al. Exposure time of enamel and dentine to saliva for protection against erosion: a study in vitro. Caries Res 2006;40(3):213–7.
63. Attin T, Knofel S, Buchalla W, et al. In situ evaluation of different remineralization periods to decrease brushing abrasion of demineralized enamel. Caries Res 2001;35(3):216–22.
64. Eisenburger M, Addy M, Hughes JA, et al. Effect of time on the remineralisation of enamel by synthetic saliva after citric acid erosion. Caries Res 2001; 35(3):211–5.
65. Lussi J, Salzmann D, Lussi A. Influence of human saliva on toothbrush abrasion of softened enamel in vitro [abstract 159]. In: Abstracts of the 56th ORCA congress. Budapest, Hungary: 2009. p. 236.
66. Joiner J, Schwarz A, Philpotts CJ, et al. The protective nature of pellicle towards toothpaste abrasion on enamel and dentine. J Dent 2008;36(5):360–8.
67. Yip HK, Smales RJ, Kaidonis JA. Management of tooth tissue loss from erosion. Quintessence Int 2002;33(7):516–20.
68. Dahl BL, Krogstad O. The effect of a partial bite raising splint on the occlusal face height. An x-ray cephalometric study in human adults. Acta Odontol Scand 1982; 40(1):17–24.
69. Bartlett DW. The role of erosion in tooth wear: aetiology, prevention and management. Int Dent J 2005;55(4):277–84.
70. Soderholm KJ, Richards ND. Wear resistance of composites: a solved problem? Gen Dent 1998;46(3):256–63.
71. Gaengler P, Hoyer I, Montag R. Clinical evaluation of posterior composite restorations: the 10-year report. J Adhes Dent 2001;3(2):185–94.
72. Manhart J, Garcia-Godoy F, Hickel R. Direct posterior restorations: clinical results and new developments. Dent Clin North Am 2002;46(2):303–39.
73. Hastings JH. Conservative restoration of function and aesthetics in a bulimic patient: a case report. Pract Periodontics Aesthet Dent 1996;8(8):729–36.
74. Tepper SA, Schmidlin PR. Technique of direct vertical bite reconstruction with composite and a splint as template. Schweiz Monatsschr Zahnmed 2005; 115(1):35–47.
75. Turssi CP, Hara AT, Serra MC, et al. Effect of storage media upon the surface micromorphology of resin-based restorative materials. J Oral Rehabil 2002; 29(9):864–71.
76. Tsuchiya S, Nikaido T, Sonoda H, et al. Ultrastructure of the dentin-adhesive interface after acid-base challenge. J Adhes Dent 2004;6(3):183–90.
77. Gomec Y, Dorter C, Ersev H, et al. Effects of dietary acids on surface microhardness of various tooth-colored restoratives. Dent Mater J 2004;23(3):429–35.

78. Aliping-McKenzie M, Linden RW, Nicholson JW. The effect of Coca-Cola and fruit juices on the surface hardness of glass-ionomers and "compomers". J Oral Rehabil 2004;31(11):1046–52.
79. Yap AU, Lim LY, Yang TY, et al. Influence of dietary solvents on strength of nanofill and ormocer composites. Oper Dent 2005;30(1):129–33.
80. Mohamed-Tahir MA, Tan HY, Woo AA, et al. Effects of pH on the microhardness of resin-based restorative materials. Oper Dent 2005;30(5):661–6.

Index

Note: Page numbers of article titles are in **boldface** type.

A

Abfraction, 430
Abrasion, 430
Antibacterial agents, topical application of, in caries, 530–533
Attrition, 430

B

Baby bottle syndrome, 433–434
Bleaching, dental, effects on enamel and dentin, 461–462
Brown-spot lesion, 431

C

Calcium-based strategies, for caries prevention, 518–519
Calculus crystals, 471–472
Caries, active, 432
    fluoride regimen in, 515
  activity assessment of, 479–480
    Nyvad's system for, 483–484
    saliva diagnostics in, 530
  advanced, restoration over soft dentin, 546
  and oral health, microbiology and role of dental plaque biofilms in, **441–454**
  and plaque, 443–451
  antimicrobial and antiseptic approaches to, 530
    limitations of, 533–534
  arrest of, natural process and, 510
  arrested or inactive, 432
  balance/imbalance model of, 495
  chemistry of, **469–478**
  clinical intervention protocols in, 500–501, 502
  complex carbohydrates and, 459
  control by nonoperative treatments, 542
  control of, sample patient letters/recommendations for, 503–505
  conventional removal of, 544
  current management approaches in, 509
  dental plaque and, 443–451
    historical perspective on, 444
    plaque bacteria in, 447
  detection activity assessment and diagnosis of, **479–493**
  detection of, concept of, 426, 434
    electronic caries monitor for, 487

Dent Clin N Am 54 (2010) 579–585
doi:10.1016/S0011-8532(10)00049-2
0011-8532/10/$ – see front matter © 2010 Elsevier Inc. All rights reserved.

Moving?

Make sure your subscription moves with you!

To notify us of your new address, find your **Clinics Account Number** (located on your mailing label above your name), and contact customer service at:

Email: **journalscustomerservice-usa@elsevier.com**

800-654-2452 (subscribers in the U.S. & Canada)
314-447-8871 (subscribers outside of the U.S. & Canada)

Fax number: 314-447-8029

Elsevier Health Sciences Division
Subscription Customer Service
3251 Riverport Lane
Maryland Heights, MO 63043

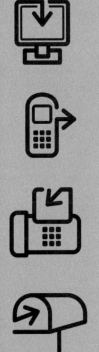

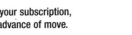

*To ensure uninterrupted delivery of your subscription,
please notify us at least 4 weeks in advance of move.